Core Competencies for Neurologists

What Clinicians Need to Know

A Report of the American Board of Psychiatry and Neurology, Inc.

Core Competencies for Neurologists

What Clinicians Need to Know

A Report of the American Board of Psychiatry and Neurology, Inc.

Edited by

Stephen C. Scheiber, M.D.
*Clinical Professor of Psychiatry, Northwestern University Medical School,
Evanston; Clinical Professor of Psychiatry, Medical College of
Wisconsin, Milwaukee; Executive Vice President,
American Board of Psychiatry and Neurology, Deerfield, Illinois*

Thomas A. M. Kramer, M.D.
*Director, Student Counseling and Resource Service,
The University of Chicago*

Susan E. Adamowski, Ed.D.
*Director, New Assessment Initiatives, American Board of Psychiatry and
Neurology, Deerfield, Illinois*

Foreword by

David C. Leach, M.D.
*Executive Director, Accreditation Council for Graduate Medical Education,
Chicago, Illinois*

With Seven Contributing Authors

Butterworth-Heinemann
An imprint of Elsevier

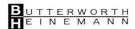

Butterworth-Heinemann is an imprint of Elsevier

Core Competencies for Neurologists   ISBN 0-7506-7465-2
First Edition

NOTICE

Medicine is an ever-changing field. Standard safety precautions must be followed but as new research and clinical experience broaden our knowledge, changes in treatment and drug therapy may become necessary or appropriate. Readers are advised to check the most current product information provided by the manufacturer of each drug to be administered to verify the recommended dose, the method and duration of administration, and contraindications. It is the responsibility of the treating physician, relying on experience and knowledge of the patient, to determine dosages and the best treatment for each individual patient. Neither the publisher nor the author assumes any liability for any injury and/or damage to persons or property arising from this publication.

♾ Recognizing the importance of preserving what has been written, Elsevier Science prints its books on acid-free paper whenever possible.

Library of Congress Cataloging-in-Publication Data

Invitational Core Competencies Conference (2001: Toronto, Ont.)
  Core competencies for neurologists: what clinicians need to know: a report of the American Board of Psychiatry and Neurology/edited by Stephen C. Scheiber, Thomas A.M. Kramer, Susan E. Adamowski; foreword by David Leach; with seven contributing authors.–1st ed.
    p. ; cm.
  Includes index.
  ISBN 0-7506-7465-2
  1. Neurology–Standards–Congresses. I. Scheiber, Stephen C. II. Kramer, Thomas A.M., 1957–III. Adamowski, Susan E., 1944–IV. American Board of Psychiatry and Neurology. V. Title.
  [DNLM: 1. Clinical Competence–standards–Congresses. 2. Neurology–standards–Congresses. WL 21 I62c 2003]
  RC346.I585 2001
  616.8–dc21   2003040352

Editor: Susan F. Pioli
Editorial Assistant: Joan Ryan

Printed in the United States of America

Last digit is the print number: 10 9 8 7 6 5 4 3 2 1

Contents

SECTION **IV**
THE IMPACT OF THE CORE COMPETENCIES   119

Contributors

Susan E. Adamowski, Ed.D.
Director, New Assessment Initiatives, American Board of Psychiatry and Neurology, Deerfield, Illinois

Harold P. Adams, Jr., M.D.
Professor, Department of Neurology, University of Iowa, Carver College of Medicine, Iowa City, Iowa

José Biller, M.D., F.A.C.P.
Professor and Chairman, Department of Neurology, Indiana University School of Medicine, Indianapolis, Indiana

Michael V. Johnston, M.D.
Professor of Neurology and Pediatrics, Johns Hopkins University School of Medicine; Senior Vice President/Chief Medical Officer, Kennedy Krieger Institute, Baltimore, Maryland

H. Royden Jones Jr., M.D.
Jaime Ortiz-Patiño Chair of Neurology and Chairman, Division of Medical Specialties, Lahey Clinic, Burlington; Clinical Professor of Neurology, Harvard Medical School; and Director of Electromyography Laboratory, Children's Hospital, Boston, Massachusetts

Thomas A. M. Kramer, M.D.
Director, Student Counseling and Resource Service, The University of Chicago

Nadia Z. Mikhael, M.D., F.R.C.P.C., F.C.A.P.
Director of Education, Royal College of Physicians and Surgeons of Canada, Ottawa, Ontario, Canada

Alan K. Percy, M.D.
William Bew White, Jr. Professor of Pediatrics, Neurology, and Neurobiology, University of Alabama at Birmingham, Birmingham, Alabama

Stephen C. Scheiber, M.D.
Clinical Professor of Psychiatry, Northwestern University Medical School, Evanston; Clinical Professor of Psychiatry, Medical College of Wisconsin, Milwaukee; Executive Vice President, American Board of Psychiatry and Neurology, Deerfield, Illinois

Nicholas A. Vick, M.D.
Professor of Neurology, Northwestern University Medical School; Chairman, Department of Neurology, Evanston Northwestern Healthcare, Evanston, Illinois

Foreword

"Success follows those adept at preserving the substance of the past by clothing it in the forms of the future. Preserve substance; modify form; know the difference."

Dee Hock
The Birth of the Chaordic Age

The substance of medicine is professional competence demonstrated through compassionate care. The Institute of Medicine (IOM) recognizes this principle in its report *Crossing the Quality Chasm* (2000), wherein it proposes ten simple rules for the twenty-first century healthcare system. The first of these rules is this: *Care is based on continuous healing relationships.* For us physicians, the delivery of competent patient care to enable healing is the essence of our professional responsibility. Continuity of that care depends to a large extent on our ability to maintain compassionate relationships with our patients. Preserving this substance is the mission of medical education.

Defining, fostering, and ensuring competence is the business of both certification and accreditation on behalf of our patients and of the profession itself. In 1999, both the Accreditation Council for Graduate Medical Education (ACGME) and the American Board of Medical Specialties (ABMS) identified organizing principles to frame our conversations about competence. These principles – Patient Care, Medical Knowledge, Interpersonal and Communication Skills, Practice-Based Learning and Improvement, Professionalism, and Systems-Based Practice – have since come to be known across the medical education continuum and across all specialties as the "general" or "core" competencies.

The recent report of the Commonwealth Fund, *Training Tomorrow's Doctors: The Medical Education Mission of Academic Health Centers* (2002) recommends that "accrediting agencies and medical professional organizations should take a leadership role in assisting [academic health centers] to develop the needs and methods to train physicians to be lifelong learners and should develop new capabilities to measure the...quality of the medical education mission." Both the ACGME and ABMS are currently engaged in identifying and developing assessment methods and tools for the competencies. We believe that this approach to the form of medical education, that is, focusing on how residents and practicing physicians demonstrate the competencies, ultimately will contribute to preserving the substance of medicine.

Nothing less than the quality of the medical education mission and ultimately, of excellent patient care, is at stake. This volume and the core competencies outlined herein provide evidence that the community of psychiatrists rises to this challenge.

David C. Leach, M.D.
Executive Director
Accreditation Council for Graduate Medical Education

Preface

This book reports on the neurology core competencies as they were discussed at the Invitational Core Competencies Conference sponsored by the American Board of Psychiatry and Neurology (ABPN) in June 2001. It attempts to document for the field of neurology what was discussed at that time in order to follow future evolutions of the core competencies. As the ABPN is the only certification Board that represents two primary specialties, we thought it appropriate to write a comparable book on core competencies for the field of psychiatry. This "sister publication" contains essentially the same material on the history of the core competency movement and on predictions for the future, but the primary content section of each book will relate directly to the specialty at hand.

It is important to note that whatever is written about core competencies is current as of its writing, but that, just as knowledge changes and grows, the listing of core competencies is in constant evolution. For the purposes of training, evaluation, and certification, particular core competencies need to be agreed upon, but core competencies as a concept have to be fluid.

During the time of the writing of this book, the core competencies outline has undergone many refinements – each after much thought and discussion. This process is expected to continue, but to become more modulated.

The Editors

Acknowledgments

Just as core competencies are not defined or assessed by any one organization or agency, the authors of this book realize that this book is the result of collaborative efforts of many individuals. As this book is primarily a report of the work of the Invitational Core Competencies Conference held in June 2001 sponsored by the American Board of Psychiatry and Neurology (ABPN), primary appreciation is due all those at the conference.

Chief among those to be acknowledged for their contributions to this book is Dr. Nadia Z. Mikhael, the Director of Education of the Royal College of Physicians and Surgeons of Canada. Dr. Mikhael served as the conference keynote speaker and a member of the reactor panel at the end of the conference. Dr. Mikhael also contributed Chapter 3 to this text. This chapter summarizes her keynote speech, outlines the *CanMEDS Report*, and provides a basic conceptual framework for organizing physician competencies.

The authors also acknowledge the others who participated in the Invitational Core Competencies Conference, especially Stanley Fahn, M.D., President of the American Academy of Neurology; Melvyn Haas, M.D., Associate Director for Medical Affairs, Substance Abuse and Medical Services Administration; David Leach, M.D., Executive Director, Accreditation Council for Graduate Medical Education; and David Nahrwold, M.D., then President-Elect of the American Board of Medical Specialties; all of whom served, along with Dr. Mikhael, as members of a reactor panel at the end of the conference.

All of the conference participants are thanked for their enthusiasm for thinking "out of the box" and for their insightful comments regarding the developing concept of core competencies.

The authors also owe a debt of gratitude to the many who contributed to and supported the beginning work on core competencies through the Accreditation Council on Graduate Medical Education and the American Board of Medical Specialties. Special thanks go to the writers of the neurology quadrad outline.

The authors would also like to acknowledge the contributions and support of all the Directors of the ABPN, without whom none of our work would be possible.

Last, but certainly not least, the authors wish to thank Shel Cappellano and Megan Thiede, the patient administrative assistants who cheerfully worked through iteration after iteration of this manuscript.

Just as the core competencies are (and will continue to be) the result of the collaborative efforts of many, this book also represents the thoughts, discussions, and writings of many others. To all of these persons, the authors are extremely grateful.

Abbreviations

360-degree evaluations	evaluations done by multiple people in a person's sphere of influence, usually superiors, peers, subordinates, and patients and their families
AAN	American Academy of Neurology
ABMS	American Board of Medical Specialties
ABPN	American Board of Psychiatry and Neurology, Inc.
ACGME	Accreditation Council for Graduate Medical Education
ACOG	American Board of Obstetrics and Gynecology
AIDS	acquired immunodeficiency syndrome
AMA	American Medical Association
ANA	American Neurological Association
angio	angiography
APA	American Psychiatric Association
CanMEDS	*Skills for the New Millennium: Report of the Societal Needs Working Group – The CanMEDS 2000 Project*
CME	continuing medical education
CSA	clinical skills assessment
CSF	cerebrospinal fluid
CT	computed tomography
D.O.	Doctor of Osteopathy
ECFMG	Educational Commission for Foreign Medical Graduates
Ed.D.	Doctor of Education
EEG	electroencephalogram/electroencephalography
EFPO	*Educating Future Physicians for Ontario Project*
EMG	electromyogram
FITER	Final In-Training (residency) Evaluation Reports
IMG	international medical graduates
MS	multiple sclerosis
M.D.	Doctor of Medicine
MCQ	multiple-choice question
MG	myasthenia gravis
MOC	maintenance of certification

MRA	magnetic resonance angiography
MRI	magnetic resonance imaging
MRS	magnetic resonance spectroscopy
MRV	magnetic resonance venography
NBME	National Board of Medical Examiners
OSCE	objective-structured clinical examination
Part I	ABPN written certification examination
Part II	ABPN oral certification examination
PDM	phenomenology, diagnosis and management of competency
PET	positron emission tomography
RCPSC	Royal College of Physicians and Surgeons of Canada (Royal College)
RRC	Residency Review Committee
SAQ	short-answer questions
SNWG	Societal Needs Working Group
SPECT	single photon emission computed tomography
TIA	transient ischemic attack
U.S.	United States

SECTION I

An Introduction to Core Competencies

The term "core competencies" is self-explanatory; core competencies are those skills and abilities that are central to, or "at the core" of, a given field. In a medical specialty, core competencies represent what physician specialists should be able to do in order to be considered minimally competent in their fields. By their very nature, core competencies are nonnegotiable.

Core competencies grew out of the focus on educational outcomes spearheaded by the U.S. Department of Education in the 1980s. The Department mandated outcome measures for all educational projects, including those involving accreditation. Heavily funded medical education systems were a prime target of this initiative and were called upon to provide evidence of responsible stewardship in preparing competent physicians to meet public healthcare needs.

From the 1980s to the present time, the interest in assessing competence has increased, and medical leaders clearly understand that unless they begin a comprehensive assessment of their own field, an outside agency is likely to conduct the assessment for them. Pressure from insurance carriers and other third parties has also intensified the effort to determine medical competence according to an objective standard.

Efforts in the United States to determine the core competencies of medical specialty fields have been led by the Accreditation Council for Graduate Medical Education (ACGME) and the American Board of Medical Specialties (ABMS). Their efforts will have an impact on medical residents and medical specialists in all fields.

This book is an attempt to explain what is happening in the field with neurology core competencies and how the competencies will affect neurology residents and practicing neurologists. Chapter 1 of this section will speak directly to that issue, underscoring the fact that both educational and practice arenas are changing rapidly. Chapter 2 will provide an historical context for the core competencies by tracing the evolving concept of medical competence in the practice of neurology from the beginning of the movement of specialty education in the late 1920s and early 1930s to the present time.

Medical competence is not a new concept, but its current iteration in the form of core competencies will change both medical education and medical practice. It is imperative that those who work as and with neurologists understand core competencies in their broadest context and their most narrow application.

1

What Core Competencies Mean to Neurologists and Trainees

Stephen C. Scheiber, M.D. and Thomas A. M. Kramer, M.D.

The practice of medicine has changed dramatically during the past few decades. Not only have medical advances altered patient care, but the societal framework of which medical care is a part has also changed drastically. Along with the growth in the sheer quantity of medical knowledge has been the popularization of that knowledge through a variety of sources. Medical television programs have always been popular. Television has more recently provided behind-the-scenes looks at physicians as real people, and not medical gods.

Patients today are more aware of health and healthcare issues than their parents and grandparents were. They are more likely to ask their physicians perceptive questions after having read about medical topics and procedures in the popular press and on the Internet. Patients demand more of their physicians today. No longer are physicians revered. Today's physician is no longer the total decision-maker when it comes to medical issues. Modern physicians are often seen as the primary experts in terms of medical knowledge, but also as partners with the patients and their families in making healthcare decisions.

With the growth of medical knowledge and the increasing astuteness of patients, demands for specialty medical services have escalated in the recent past. Insurance companies and other third-party payers have not been pleased with this. In order to stem the rising tide of insurance claims, managed care companies are making healthcare decisions, often serving as gatekeepers for those in various insurance programs. Decisions made in the managed care office often determine what medical care a patient will ultimately receive. Not only do managed care companies determine the type and level of care for which insurance will pay, but the managed care companies also often determine who can deliver that care. Very often physicians who are not Board-certified are dismissed as being inadequate providers of care. Today more than ever, medical credentials and not just the medical degree determine how busy physicians are and what their income will be.

These changes in the medical care scene could be positive. Patients should be receiving the best care available, according to their needs, from the most qualified

3

physicians. In practice, this is not always the case. What can be said with assurance, however, is that physicians today are being held more accountable than ever before for their knowledge, skills, and attitudes. Medical competence, once assumed because physicians had "M.D." or a "D.O." following their names, has been called into question.

Competence is not an all-or-nothing proposition. Competence is measured along a sliding scale through demonstrated knowledge and performed tasks. Competence is assessed by degrees. The measuring of medical competence has been a difficult activity. Just how much and exactly what must a physician know and be able to do to be judged "competent?" Different groups have tackled these questions and listed the knowledge, skills, and attitudes that must be demonstrated by physicians to demonstrate competence. Some of these groups include the following:

- The American Board of Medical Specialties (ABMS) Task Force on Competence
- The Accreditation Council for Graduate Medical Education (ACGME) Outcome Project Advisory Group
- The Association of American Medical Colleges' Medical School Objectives Project Group
- The Federated Council for Internal Medicine Task Force on the Internal Medicine Residency Curriculum
- The National Association for Competency Assurance
- The Pew Health Professions Commission

Various groups have recently gotten together to agree on categories of "core competencies." Core competencies are just what their name implies. They are "competencies" or abilities that are "core" or central to medical practice. Core competencies are nonnegotiable. Some core competencies are essentially uniform across specialties and subspecialties; others are, by necessity, specialty-specific.

This book will lay out in some detail what the core competencies might be for the field of neurology, how they came into being and, most importantly, how they might affect practicing neurologists and those who hope to become so. The first section of the book will set the stage for the current concept of physician "competence" by explaining the logic of the development of the current thought. Section II will provide two different views of how to look at core competencies: what the leaders in Canada have done and, based on some of their work, what is currently being done in the United States.

Section III will discuss specific core competencies as currently delineated for neurologists across the six core competency categories agreed upon by the ACGME and the ABMS. These categories include Patient Care, Medical Knowledge, Interpersonal and Communications Skills, Practice-Based Learning and Improvement, Professionalism, and Systems-Based Practice. Section III will also include discussions of when in a physician's career these competencies should be assessed and what methodologies would be appropriate for those assessments. Throughout this section of the book, it will be clear that core competencies are "living entities;" they will constantly be in development and under refinement. These development and refinement processes will not be the purview of any one organization or agency, but will rather reflect the input of medical school faculty, residency training directors, practitioners in the field, individual specialty Boards, specialty societies, the ACGME, the ABMS, and others with an interest in the field.

Section IV will conclude the book by discussing how the neurology core competencies are changing Board certification and recertification. This section will also discuss changes medical school faculty and residency training directors will likely have to make and how practicing neurologists will likely have to change behaviors to maintain their Board certification.

2

The Evolving Concept of Clinical Competence in Neurology Practice

Stephen C. Scheiber, M.D. and Thomas A. M. Kramer, M.D.

Today, with the American Board of Medical Specialties (ABMS) serving as the umbrella organization of 24 separate specialty Boards, one hears of medical competence discussed in terms of certification, recertification and, most recently, maintenance of certification. It is helpful to remember that these aspects of competence – becoming certified initially, getting certified again or repeatedly, and continuously maintaining certification – are evolving views of the same basic idea, namely, that medical specialists should be held to certain educational and performance standards in order to practice their specialties.

The practice of medical specialties can be documented to before the twentieth century, but it was not until the late 1920s and early 1930s that the specialty movement gained real momentum in the United States. This was the result of scientific and technical advances, which brought attendant increases in specialized medical knowledge. In addition, independent specialty departments were beginning to be formed in medical schools, which were greatly expanded after World War II. As part of the independent departments, there was an increasing emphasis on research and how it applied to the expanding knowledge base for the specialties. This subsequently led to greater differentiation among the specialties. Developing urban areas also provided concentrations of people who could support medical specialists.

The issue for neurologists, as well as all other medical specialists, was to gain public recognition for their specialties. This recognition was based on both altruistic reasons and professional survival. The patient, or in aggregate, "the public," deserved the best medical care possible. Providing such care is the undeniable altruistic aim of all medical practitioners, including medical specialists.

Specialists, however, sensed that both professional and financial gains could be achieved if their professions were regulated from within. It would benefit the competent, well-trained specialists to have themselves identified as such and keep those with lesser capabilities outside their medical specialty field. Thus, specialty Boards began organizing formally: the American Board of Ophthalmology in

1916, the American Board of Otolaryngology in 1924, the American Board of Obstetrics and Gynecology in 1930, and the forerunner of today's American Board of Dermatology in 1930.

The impetus for increased zeal to form a certification body was fueled by both professional and practical concerns. There was a desire for professional recognition of the specialties, but there was also a growing concern that if the professions did not regulate themselves from within, then external agencies would step in to handle that task. There was generalized concern that the American Medical Association (AMA), the state medical societies, the National Board of Medical Examiners (NBME), or some combination of these groups would define competence in psychiatry. J. V. May, M.D., in his presidential address to the American Psychiatric Association (APA) in 1933 stated:

> "It will at least be conceded, I think, that if we are to maintain a position of supremacy in our own field, we must establish standards fully equivalent to those already erected by the surgeons, internists, ophthalmologists, otolaryngologists, obstetricians and gynecologists, dermatologists, and pediatrists." (May 1933, p. 14)

In June 1933, the Section on Nervous and Mental Diseases of the AMA resolved that it would cooperate with the APA, the American Neurological Association (ANA) and other concerned national organizations in forming a certification Board to discuss the formation of a joint certification board for neurology and psychiatry. "The inclusion of neurology [with psychiatry] was in keeping with the stand taken by the Council on Medical Education and Hospitals of the AMA, a stand that favored a single Board when fields overlap to the extent that neurology and psychiatry overlap" (Hollender 1991, p. 4). Ground rules were agreed upon at this first meeting that are still basically in effect today. These rules had to do with representation on the Board, separate qualifications being required for each specialty, and the fact that a candidate who wished to be certified in both specialties had to demonstrate high proficiency in both areas.

The second meeting of the combined group on April 14, 1934, with Adolf Meyer, M.D., presiding, yielded agreement on the outline of prerequisites for examination and certification. These included that all prospective candidates should: (1) be graduates of approved medical schools and possess a license to practice medicine; (2) have served a general internship; (3) be recognized as ethical practitioners in their communities; and (4) be members of the AMA (with exceptions made for Canadians). Experiential prerequisites varied by specialty.

In 1934, *Regulations for the Guidance of the Board of Certification in Psychiatry and Neurology in Establishing the Requirement for Such Certificates* discussed separate certifying examinations for neurology and psychiatry. The document stated that:

> "The examinations both written and practical are proposed to test the ability of the candidates to meet the situations to which they might at any time be subjected. They [the examinations] will be of such a type that no adequately trained individual will fail to pass, and they will be sufficiently searching so that the specialist in fact may be separated from the specialist in name. They will be held one or more times a year."

The document further stated that:

"Practical examinations will include the examination of patients under the supervision of an examiner, the identification of specimens in the laboratory of anatomy and pathology and the interpretation of roentgenograms, but will not require the performance of diagnostic tests properly in the field of laboratory medicine. The manner of examining both neurological and psychiatric cases and the reasoning and deductions therefrom constitute the most important part of the whole examination." (see Note 1)

Of the first organizational meeting of the Board being held on October 20, 1934, with Adolf Meyer, M.D., as chairman, it can be said that the first official core competencies for certification in neurology and psychiatry became operationalized. The Board offered three types of certification: in neurology; in psychiatry; or in both. Physicians desiring to be "double-Boarded" had to meet the requirements for and pass the examination in both specialties. The first certification examination was administered in Philadelphia on June 7, 1935.

While neurology and psychiatry were to be seen as distinct specialties, all candidates took the same examination from 1935 through 1946. The difference between the two specialties was evidenced by different scoring standards. These scoring differences came to be known as the "major" and the "minor" examinations. For a candidate in neurology, the "major examination" referred to the neurology questions on the exam, while the "minor examination" referred to the psychiatry questions on the exam. (For a psychiatry candidate, this was reversed.) A higher score was required on the major examination, but candidates also had to pass the minor examination. Physicians seeking "double-Boarding" had to meet the requirements for major examinations in both specialties.

From its inception, the ABPN focused almost exclusively on the development and administration of certifying examinations to denote competence within the specialties of neurology and psychiatry. Part of the issue of competence involved setting standards to determine who would be allowed to take the certification examination. Qualifications for examination eligibility in the early days of the exam included graduation from medical school, one year of internship training, plus specialty training and clinical experience for specified amounts of time. The Board also attempted to establish ethical and professional standards of conduct as examination prerequisites, but these proved to be unworkable. Thus, early Board certification communicated to the public that the successful candidate had fulfilled educational and experiential requirements and had passed an examination, but were essentially silent on issues of ethics and professional conduct.

ISSUES OF BEING A DUAL BOARD

Certification within a dual Board raises many questions. One of the main reasons that neurology and psychiatry formed one Board for certification purposes had to do with the politics of the time. The AMA Council on Medical Education and Hospitals and the Advisory Board of Medical Specialties (the forerunner of the ABMS) encouraged complementary specialties to unite as one Board simply to stem the proliferation of Boards. This was done, for example, with obstetrics and gynecology, which formed one Board in 1930, and with dermatology and syphilology, which formed one Board in 1932. When differences between two areas could not be overcome, two separate Boards were created. This was the case with the formation of the American Board of Ophthalmology in 1916 and the American Board of Otolaryngology in 1924.

Besides the push of politics to incorporate as one Board, the practical matter of the number of neurologists had to be considered. "At the time of the inception of the ABPN, there were not enough neurologists to justify the establishment of an examining Board in neurology" (Forster 1960, as quoted in Hollender 1991). Thus, for both political and practical reasons the medical fields of neurology and psychiatry decided to unite under one Board. In December 1933, egalitarian minds prevailed in deciding, despite the preponderance in terms of numbers of psychiatrists over neurologists, that there should be equal representation of both specialties on the board. At the same time, however, decisions were made that qualifications, examinations, and certifications would be separate for the two medical specialties. Those wishing to be certified in both specialties would have to qualify for both examinations. While the Board did encourage dual certification, no concessions were made in reducing the number of years of education and experience in each field to make this a more manageable accomplishment. In addition, as stated earlier, physicians desiring "double-Boarding" had to achieve scores equivalent to the major areas for both neurology and psychiatry on the examination; there was no major/minor difference for these candidates.

Through the years, there have been many points of contention between neurologists and psychiatrists, even over such things as the name of the Board. The neurologists claimed that the name should have been the American Board of Neurology and Psychiatry, with the names of the two specialties in alphabetical order. The psychiatrists claimed that their greater numbers should give their specialty first berth in the Board's name. In the end, the psychiatrists prevailed, and the American Board of Psychiatry and Neurology was incorporated in 1934.

The work of the Board was to establish standards of competence for the medical fields of neurology and psychiatry. Over the years, changes in the qualifications for and nature of the examinations separated the two fields even more than they had been separated initially. This separation can be documented by studying the *Information for Applicants* booklets, which were revised almost annually, as they changed over the years.

The earliest available *Information for Applicants* booklet is the fourth edition from 1939. Unfortunately, the first through third editions are not available. The fourth edition booklet states that the ABPN was created "in response to a widespread desire among specialists in psychiatry and neurology for some means of distinguishing the fully qualified specialist from the would-be specialist of inferior training and inadequate training." This statement was later amended to read, "This action [of creating the ABPN] was taken as a method of identifying the qualified specialists in Psychiatry and Neurology" (Hollender 1991, p. 29). In all cases, the *Information for Applicants* booklet stressed that the main goal of the ABPN was to separate the competent from the incompetent in the practice of neurology and psychiatry.

The 1939 edition of the *Information for Applicants* booklet describes in some detail how competence was judged. It stated that:

> "The same examination is given whether a candidate applies for certification in psychiatry or in neurology or in both psychiatry and neurology. The Board requires some proficiency in neurology on the part of those it certifies in psychiatry and vice versa, but judges the candidate in accordance with the certificate he seeks."

It is interesting to note that the early certification examinations were almost entirely oral. According to the 1939 *Information for Applicants* booklet, besides an identification and discussion of the functions of the more important anatomic structures of the brain and spinal cord, a discussion of gross and microscopic pathologic specimens, and the interpretation of roentgenograms dealing with neurological disorders, two hours were devoted to an oral examination on the subjects of psychobiology and psychopathology. The candidate was also required to examine four patients, two with neurological and two with psychiatric disorders, and to discuss patient findings with the examiners. The *Information for Applicants* booklet clearly states that the patient examinations, each of which lasted about an hour, were the most important parts of the examination. In addition, the 1939 edition states that "some acquaintance with the history of psychiatry and neurology, with the body of the doctrine, and with recent advances is presupposed." These areas of knowledge were also addressed on the oral examination.

Not all practicing neurologists and psychiatrists of the time were required to take the certification examination to demonstrate their competence. Some more senior members of the professions were "grandfathered" into certification. To be considered for grandfathering, a candidate had to have graduated from medical school in or before 1919, to have specialized in neurology and/or psychiatry for at least fifteen years, and to have a satisfactory professional record.

The first cohort of examinees sat for the certification examination at the Philadelphia General Hospital on June 7, 1935. Of the 31 candidates, 21 passed the examination (two in neurology alone, ten in psychiatry alone, and nine in both neurology and psychiatry). Essay-type questions piloted with this examination were judged unsuccessful and thus eliminated.

The ABPN certification examination continued in the above format until 1946. The only notable change was the introduction of true–false questions in 1943 but, like the earlier essay questions, these were deemed unsatisfactory.

Changes in the 1946 examination highlighted changes in the certification process that have continued and increased during the years. Not only were separate examinations for neurology and psychiatry given in 1946, but the emphasis in each exam shifted. Previously, the joint examination had devoted approximately three hours each to neurology and psychiatry. In 1946, the emphasis was shifted to devote four hours to the major specialty of the candidate and two hours to the minor specialty.

Perhaps even more importantly, the 1946 *Information for Applicants* booklet stressed that competence in dealing with patients and not just factual knowledge was the main objective in the examination process. This is clearly shown in the expanded section on requirements for training as a prerequisite for the examination. The 1946 edition of the *Information for Applicants* booklet stated for the first time: "Oral and practical examinations will be given in the basic sciences with special regard to their clinical implications."

The previous sentence was repeated year after year. In 1949, a new sentence followed that one: "Written examinations *may be given* at the discretion of the Board." In 1966, that statement was amended to read: "Written examinations *will be given* at the discretion of the Board." (Italics not in original.)

THE DEVELOPMENT OF THE WRITTEN PORTION OF THE CERTIFICATION EXAMINATION

In 1949, according to the minutes of a policy meeting, the directors of the ABPN also began in earnest to develop a written examination. Each director was to send ten suitable multiple-choice questions for use in the development of separate written neurology and psychiatry examinations. Not enough usable questions were received, however, and discussion of the creation of a written competency examination occurred at the next three policy meetings. Then "the whole idea was dropped because the directors could not agree on the questions, to say nothing of the answers" (Hollender 1991, p. 32).

The potential written examination was seen alternately as a screening device to deselect unqualified candidates and as a part of the examination itself. Efforts to create a written examination in each of the medical specialties occurred sporadically during the 1950s and early 1960s. By 1963, the need for a written examination seemed to become a practical necessity. A written examination would serve two major purposes: (1) it might eliminate or at least lessen reliability problems with the oral examinations; and (2) it could help to cope with the ever-increasing number of candidates seeking to take the examination. Consensus now seemed to favor using the written examination as a screening tool for admitting qualified candidates to the oral examinations.

Having been unsuccessful in creating a written examination themselves, the directors of the ABPN turned to the National Board of Medical Examiners (NBME) for assistance, and in 1966 the first written examination was given. Initially, it was thought that the written examination could be administered immediately preceding the oral examination, but for test security purposes, several different versions of the examination would be required. These examination versions would require a substantially larger test item pool than was currently available, and therefore, it was decided that the written portion of the certification examination would be administered separately from the oral examination and only one time per year. This written examination increased in length from two to three hours and came to be known as Part I of the two-part ABPN certification examination. This written examination was administered for the first time in 1967, and only those successful on this examination could register for the oral examination. Labeling the written examination as Part I and the oral examination as Part II legitimized the former as a required part of the certification examination, and not merely a screening tool. It continued to provide a screening function, however, in that its successful completion was a prerequisite for the oral (Part II) examination.

From the beginning of the administration of the written examination, the directors of the ABPN took this part of competency testing very seriously. Instead of merely relying on the NBME to create the written examination, the ABPN recruited practicing specialists to develop questions for their own question pool. The ABPN *Annual Report for 1969* stated that:

> "The written examination is considered to be essentially a method to determine the candidate's fund of knowledge. The principal purpose of the oral examination is to provide the candidate with the opportunity to apply his knowledge and thereby demonstrate his clinical competence."

Besides being used as a prerequisite for admission to the oral examination, the written examination also changed the format of the oral examination by being able to assess adequately the general knowledge of the basic sciences. Thus, the oral examination was reduced in time and devoted toward the clinical application of basic knowledge. Oral examination sections in basic psychiatry for neurologists and in basic neurology for psychiatrists were also eliminated.

For a time, a bridging committee was established to identify basic sciences common to both neurology and psychiatry, but after a few years it was determined that two separate committees – one for basic sciences in neurology and one for basic sciences in psychiatry – needed to be established. These committees focused their efforts on the written examinations.

In 1970, the written portion of the ABPN certification examination first used pictorial material, and this was seen as a major step forward in the developing sophistication of the examination.

In 1975, the section of the Part I examination that tested both basic neurology and basic psychiatry – the only common portion of the examination for the two specialties – was replaced by two separate examinations. Thus, the neurology and psychiatry certification examinations could be seen as completely different entities.

OTHER EVOLUTIONS IN THE ABPN CERTIFICATION EXAMINATION

Increasing numbers of candidates to be examined for Part II of the examination called for increasing numbers of patients, increasing numbers of examiners, and increasing numbers of clinical sites for testing. Clearly, a new venue had to be found to accomplish the same competency testing purposes.

The use of motion pictures for some sessions of patient contact was discussed, but never pursued because of the costs involved. When lower-cost audiovisual tapes became available, they were assessed for use in the late 1970s. Studies showed a high level of concurrence on the part of the candidates between the use of live patients and their videotaped counterparts (Greenblatt 1977, as reported in Hollender 1991). By the beginning of the 1982 examination cycle, the Part II examination in psychiatry was comprised of a one-hour interview of a live patient (including half an hour of discussion about the candidate's examination of the patient) and a one-hour videotaped presentation of a patient (including half an hour of discussion of the candidate's analysis of the videotape). Both the live patient interview and its videotaped counterpart were deemed more effective at testing complex interpersonal skills than could be assessed using any written examination (Small 1980). With the live patient interview, these skills included assessing how the candidate related to the patient, how the clinical interview was conducted, and the ability to organize and present data in the form of a differential diagnosis and medical treatment plan. The videotaped portion of the examination focused on the synthesis of the data presented, the differential diagnosis, and the formulation of a treatment plan.

At the same time, the neurology oral examination became a three-hour process with one hour devoted to a patient examination and two hours to vignettes. Neurologists believed that videotapes were not suitable for their purposes and used patient vignettes (short descriptions of patients complete with clinical findings) as stimuli for the non-patient portion of the examination. Examination of an actual patient remained key to both neurology and psychiatry oral (Part II) examinations.

The ABPN examinations in neurology and psychiatry, which had begun as a single examination, were now two completely separate examinations. While each examination tested for competency in both subject areas, each focused clearly on its own "major" area. By the 1980s, not only were the examinations completely separate, but the grading sessions for them were also separate.

SUMMARY AND CONCLUSION

From its inception, the ABPN was devoted to assessing the competence of neurologists and psychiatrists for the ultimate benefits of the patients they served. Various testing formats were used over the years. These became increasingly specialty-specific and matured through evolutions often dictated by the number of candidates needing to be served.

The commitment of the ABPN to use the six categories of core competencies adopted by the Accreditation Council for Graduate Medical Education (ACGME) and the ABMS represents a continued step in the evolution of sophistication in the measurement of physician competence. This step, like the many that preceded it, will provide challenges in its implementation, but will ultimately enhance the assessment of physician competence.

NOTES

1. The full document can be found in Hollender, M.H.: The founding of the ABPN. In: *The American Board of Psychiatry and Neurology: The First Fifty Years*. Edited by M.H. Hollender. Deerfield, IL: ABPN pp. 12–14, 1991.

REFERENCES

Greenblatt M. *History of Significance of Recent Rulings of the ABPN*. Paper presented at the Annual Meeting of the American Psychiatric Association, Toronto, Ontario, Canada, May 2–6, 1977.

Hollender MH. The examination in psychiatry. In: *The American Board of Psychiatry and Neurology: The First Fifty Years*. Edited by Hollender MH. Deerfield, IL: American Board of Psychiatry and Neurology, 1991, p. 34.

Hollender MH. The founding of the ABPN. In: *The American Board of Psychiatry and Neurology: The First Fifty Years*. Edited by Hollender MH. Deerfield, IL: American Board of Psychiatry and Neurology, 1991, p. 4.

May JV. The establishment of psychiatric standards by the association. Am J Psychiatry 1933;90:1–15.

Meyer A. Presidential address: thirty-five years of psychiatry in the United States and our present outlook. Am J Psychiatry 1928;85:1–31.

Small SM. Role of objective examinations in psychiatry. In: *Comprehensive Textbook of Psychiatry/III*, 3rd Edition. Edited by Kaplan HI, Freedman AM, Sadock BJ. Baltimore, MD: Williams & Wilkins, 1980, pp. 2974–2975.

Origins of Core Competencies: Canadian Groundbreaking and American Development

As Section I of this book has shown, the concept of medical competence has evolved over time. Just as with other professions, those who performed various professional tasks in the past have found their fields becoming increasingly regimented. Educational requirements are generally the first to be applied to a profession, and only much later are practice parameters established as assessment measures.

A simple example of this involves the profession of school-teaching. From the time America was first settled until the early 1900s, the teacher in each village was generally the one who had learned to read and to compute and who was not needed for other life-maintaining chores on the farm or in the home. These "standards," such as they were, sufficed and even worked well. As the general population became both more literate and numerate, many more people could have qualified to serve as teachers, except for the simple fact that other, generally more subsistence-related, work was required of them; they were required to till the fields or to weave cloth for the family's clothing.

As farm production methods required fewer workers and industrial methods reduced backbreaking housekeeping chores, one might have expected a market glut of those qualified to serve as their communities' teachers, but an interesting change came about. Educational standards for teachers were introduced, and only those with a high school diploma – later some college training – and still later, a two-year college degree were judged qualified to teach. During this time in our country, normal or teacher-training colleges abounded in order to keep pace with the need for more and more teachers as children were freed from full-time chores to be able to attend school.

Because this system seemed to work well, it became more sophisticated. Longer schooling, the mandatory four-year college diploma, was required for public school teachers. At about this same time, teacher-training also became more specialized. Someone desiring to become a teacher had to decide at the beginning of training if contact with young children or older children would be preferred, and then in the case of the older children, what particular subjects would be taught. Teacher certification was granted based on the filing of an appropriate diploma, which came to require a certain minimal amount of coursework in the methods of teaching.

Not until fairly recently have teachers been required to take minimum skills competency tests. These tests focus on acquired knowledge, but not at all on the ability to communicate that knowledge. If the content was mastered and the neophyte teachers survived a period of "practice teaching" with a more senior teacher, then that person was judged to be a teacher for evermore.

When these requirements were judged to be insufficient, teachers were forced to receive successful evaluations from their supervisors for their first two or three years of teaching in order to be granted tenure, or lifetime certification. Even with lifetime tenure, some more sophisticated school districts are requiring continuing education credits. These credits are generally earned through colleges and universities, and the teachers involved in these programs generally only have to present a grade report for continued employment and, in many cases, salary advancement. Only very recently has there been talk about higher-level and on-going competency testing, and the focus here has been again on knowledge acquisition, not knowledge sharing, which is really what teaching is.

Physicians have run a track parallel with teachers in many respects, but as the body of knowledge required of a physician is much, much larger than that required for an elementary or high school teacher, the requirements for physicians have been both more numerous and more stringent. Increasing demands have been placed on physicians in the educational arena, and certification requirements for specialized fields in medicine have been developed.

Just as with teachers, physician competence has focused more on the acquisition of knowledge and less on the skills that demonstrate the implementation of that knowledge. With greater consumer awareness and increasing problems funding medical care through third parties, the competence of physicians is under scrutiny in a way that it never before has been. With ever-increasing amounts of specialized medical knowledge – and access to that information, acquired knowledge is almost a given for any Board-certified medical specialist. While keeping up to date academically in one's specialty field is a mark of competence, new standards of competence for physicians have begun to be implemented.

Chapter 3 discusses these standards of physician competence in terms of the roles that a physician specialist must play. This concept of physician competence was developed by the Royal College of Physicians and Surgeons of Canada and includes the seven roles played by each physician: medical expert (or clinical decision-maker), communicator, collaborator, manager, health advocate, scholar, and professional. The premise on which this work rests is that while the role of being a "medical expert" or "clinical decision-maker" is central to being a specialist, competence in the other six roles is essential to success in the primary role.

Chapter 4 discusses how the Accreditation Council for Graduate Medical Education (ACGME) and the American Board of Medical Specialties (ABMS) have approached the subject of competency for physician specialists. The ACGME and ABMS have looked not at the roles a physician specialist plays, but rather at six broad areas of competence that must be mastered. These six areas include patient care, medical knowledge, interpersonal and communication skills, practice-based learning and improvement, professionalism, and systems-based practice. Competencies in each area have been delineated through a study of medical education and practice as represented by a residency program director, a representative of the Residency Review Council of the ACGME, a member of the area's specialty Board, and a resident physician. The six categories of core competencies listed above are discussed in detail in the chapters of Section III.

3

Advance Standards: The Canadian Concept of Specialty Competence as Delineated by Physician Roles

Nadia Z. Mikhael, M.D.

THE IMPORTANCE OF THE WORK ON CORE COMPETENCIES DONE IN CANADA

Some of the earliest studies performed to delineate the necessary competencies for medical specialists were carried out in Canada through the efforts of the Royal College of Physicians and Surgeons. As the keynote speaker for the ABPN Invitational Core Competencies Conference sponsored by the American Board of Psychiatry and Neurology held in Toronto in June 2001, I was pleased to share our pioneering work with my American peers. I assured the American medical leaders who had gathered for the conference that they were on the right track in listing medical specialty competencies for assessment.

THE BACKGROUND OF THE CanMEDS

The preliminary work of the core competencies in Canada is best delineated in the *CanMEDS 2000 Project Report*, a 1996 publication. The full title of the part of the *CanMEDS 2000 Project Report* that concerns core competencies is *Skills for the New Millennium: Report of the Societal Needs Working Group* (Table 3.1) (see Note 1). This report describes our attempt at the Royal College to establish guidelines for optimal specialty medical care through an analysis of the competencies needed by physicians practicing in different medical specialties. The framework for our listing of core competencies is divided by the seven roles played by each physician: medical expert (or clinical decision-maker), communicator, collaborator, manager, health advocate, scholar, and professional.

The premise on which our work rests is that while the role of being a "medical expert" or "clinical decision-maker" is central to being a specialist, competence in the other six roles is essential to success in the primary care role. All sixteen medical schools in Canada have agreed with this framework and are working to make certain that by the end of residency training, all specialists will have a grounding in each role plus the background to develop expertise as needed any time in their future careers.

In addition, work through the Royal College in the areas of accreditation, specialty-specific objectives, and evaluation has incorporated the "role framework" into all aspects of postgraduate medical education. This means that in Canada all stages of medical education from residency through professional practice are operating under the same set of expectations, one set of core competencies divided into the tasks of the seven different roles a specialist plays (see Note 2).

Our CanMEDS 2000 Project began in 1993 as an initiative of the Health and Public Policy Committee of the Royal College. The overall goal of this project was to ensure that postgraduate specialty training programs in Canada be fully responsive to societal needs. The main organizing principle of our project was to better meet the specialty medical needs of the Canadian public by changing from a supply-side (focusing on the interests of those providing medical education) to a demand-side orientation (focusing on the needs of individual patients in the context of the Canadian population at large).

One component of the CanMEDS 2000 Project was the Societal Needs Working Group (SNWG). The charge given to the SNWG was to outline the objectives and the educational and evaluation strategies for various competencies and to make recommendations for their implementation, including how these new program measures would impact accreditation of postgraduate programs and the certification of residents.

THE FRAMEWORK OF ROLES THAT A PHYSICIAN PLAYS

Our concept of the delineation of physician competencies according to roles originated with the *Educating Future Physicians for Ontario Project (EFPO)*. The SNWG realized that they had to broaden the Ontario focus of the EFPO to consider the medical needs of creating competencies for physician roles that would serve the people of the entire country. Using both published and unpublished literature – including that of consumer surveys and focus groups – the SNWG collected information on general physician competencies and then organized this information into the roles a physician plays. These roles as listed earlier are medical expert (or clinical decision-maker), communicator, collaborator, manager, health advocate, scholar, and professional, with the medical expert role being key to all.

Different task forces focused on the different roles and defined key competencies for each. To implement the role framework of physician competencies, our list of the competencies was broadened to include specific educational objectives, relevant learning points, effective evaluation measures, and pertinent faculty development issues for each role. The framework of our CanMEDS 2000 Project is therefore the product of many months' work involving medical education experts across Canada. It reflects overlapping clusters of the generic knowledge, attitudes, and skill set required of all specialists while allowing for the unique competencies of our fifty-eight different medical specialties.

Two cohorts of Royal College Fellows and all Canadian specialty program directors were selected to validate the work of the SNWG. Survey respondents were asked to rate each of the competencies from two perspectives: first, how important that competency was to their clinical practice; and second, how well they felt they had been prepared for operationalizing that competency during their training programs. Overall, it appeared that new fellows and program directors identified with each of the roles listed, but that in certain key areas training were deemed poor.

Table 3.1, which is taken from the *CanMEDS 2000 Project Report*, identifies the seven roles being played by physicians and the key competencies assigned to them. The next section of this chapter provides a more complete description of each role a physician specialist must play in order to be deemed competent.

Table 3.1 Essential Roles and Key Competencies of Specialty Physicians

Roles	Key Competencies *The physician must be able to:*
Medical Expert (a.k.a. Clinical Decision-Maker)	• Demonstrate diagnostic and therapeutic skills for ethical and effective patient care • Access and apply relevant information to clinical practice • Demonstrate effective consultation services with respect to patient care, education, and legal opinions
Communicator	• Establish therapeutic relationships with patients and their families • Obtain and synthesize relevant history from patients, their families, and their communities • Listen effectively • Discuss appropriate information with patients, their families, and the healthcare team
Collaborator	• Consult effectively with other physicians and healthcare professionals • Contribute effectively to other interdisciplinary team activities
Manager Manager (cont.)	• Utilize resources effectively to balance patient care, learning needs, and outside activities • Work effectively and efficiently in a healthcare organization • Utilize information technology to optimize patient care, life-long learning, and other activities
Health Advocate	• Identify the important determinants of health affecting patients • Contribute effectively to the improved health of patients and communities • Recognize and respond to those issues where advocacy is appropriate

(continued)

Table 3.1 Essential Roles and Key Competencies of Specialty Physicians—cont'd

Roles	Key Competencies The physician must be able to:
Scholar	• Develop, implement, and monitor a personal continuing education strategy • Critically appraise sources of medical information • Facilitate learning of patients, house staff/students, and other health professionals • Contribute to the development of new knowledge
Professional	• Deliver the highest quality care with integrity, honesty, and compassion • Exhibit appropriate personal and interpersonal professional behaviors • Practice medicine ethically consistent with the obligations of a physician

ROLE DELINEATION
The Role of Medical Expert

The role of medical expert is the central role a physician plays and draws on the competencies of all of the other roles. As delineated in the *CanMEDS 2000 Project Report*, as a medical expert, a specialist should be able to demonstrate the following competencies:

1. *Demonstrate diagnostic and therapeutic skills to effectively and ethically manage a spectrum of patient care problems within the boundaries of the specialty.* This includes the ability to do the following:
   • Elicit a relevant, concise, and accurate history.
   • Conduct an effective physical examination.
   • Carry out relevant procedures to collect, analyze, and interpret data.
   • Reach a diagnosis.
   • Perform appropriate therapeutic procedures to help resolve a patient's problem.
2. *Access and apply relevant information and therapeutic options to clinical practice.* This includes the ability to do the following:
   • Pose an appropriate patient-related question.
   • Execute a systematic search for evidence.
   • Critically evaluate medical literature and other evidence in order to optimize clinical decision-making.
3. *Demonstrate medical expertise in situations other than in direct patient care.* This includes the ability to do the following:
   • Provide testimony as an expert witness.
   • Give presentations.

4. *Recognize personal limits of expertise.* This includes the ability to do the following:
   - Decide if and when other professionals are needed to contribute to a patient's care.
   - Implement a personal program to maintain and upgrade professional medical competence.
5. *Demonstrate effective consultation skills.* This includes the ability to do the following:
   - Present well-documented patient assessments and recommendations in both verbal and written form in response to a request from another health professional.

The Role of Communicator

As a communicator, a specialist must be able to obtain information from and convey information to patients, their families, and other healthcare professionals concerned about the patients. Because obtaining and conveying such information is essential to assure humane, high-quality care of patients, the role of communicator is integral to the functioning of a medical expert. As delineated in the *CanMEDS 2000 Project Report*, as a communicator, a specialist should be able to demonstrate the following competencies:

1. *Establish therapeutic relationships with patients.* This includes the ability to do the following:
   - Establish and maintain rapport.
   - Foster an environment characterized by understanding, trust, empathy, and confidentiality.
2. *Elicit and synthesize relevant information from patients, their families, and/or their communities about patients' problems.* This includes the ability to do the following:
   - Explore patients' beliefs, concerns, and expectations about the origin, nature, and management of their illnesses.
   - Assess the impact of factors such as age, gender, ethnocultural background, social support, and emotional influences on patients' illnesses.
3. *Discuss appropriate information with patients, their families, and other healthcare providers to facilitate optimal healthcare of patients.* This includes the ability to do the following:
   - Inform and counsel patients in a sensitive and respectful manner.
   - Foster understanding, discussion, and the patients' active participation in decisions about their care.
   - Listen to patients.
   - Communicate effectively with other healthcare providers to assure optimal and consistent care of patients and their families.
   - Maintain clear, accurate, and appropriate records.

The Role of Collaborator

A medical expert does not work in isolation, but rather as a partner within a coordinated team involved in the care of a particular patient or group of patients. As a collaborator, a specialist must function well as a part of this team to ensure optimal patient care. Collaboration occurs in hospitals, practice settings, committee work, research, teaching, and learning. As delineated in the *CanMEDS 2000 Project Report*, as a collaborator, a specialist should be able to demonstrate the following competencies:

1. *Consult effectively with other physicians and healthcare professionals.* This includes the ability to do the following:
   - Develop investigations, treatments, and continuing care plans in partnership with patients and their other healthcare providers.
   - Recognize the limits of personal expertise.
   - Understand the roles and expertise of the other members of the healthcare team.
   - Inform and involve patients and their families in decision-making.
   - Integrate the opinions of patients and their caregivers into management plans.
2. *Contribute effectively to other interdisciplinary team activities.* This includes the ability to do the following:
   - Recognize team members' areas of expertise.
   - Respect the opinions and roles of individual team members.
   - Contribute to healthy team development and conflict resolution.
   - Contribute personal expertise to the teams' tasks.

The Role of Manager

Managers allocate finite healthcare and other resources in their daily practice of making decisions about time, staff, tasks, policies, and their personal lives. This involves the ability to prioritize effectively and assume the role of leader, when necessary, to execute tasks within the healthcare team. In the role of manager, a medical expert often finds himself/herself as the formal or informal leader of the healthcare team. As delineated in the *CanMEDS 2000 Project Report*, as a manager, a specialist should be able to demonstrate the following competencies:

1. *Utilize time and resources effectively in order to balance patient care, learning needs, outside activities, and personal life.* This includes the ability to do the following:
   - Employ effective time management and self-assessment skills to formulate realistic expectations and a balanced lifestyle.
2. *Allocate finite healthcare and health education resources effectively.* This includes the ability to do the following:
   - Make sound judgments on resource allocation based on evidence of the benefit to individual patients and the population served.

3. *Work effectively and efficiently in a healthcare organization.* This includes the ability to do the following:
   - Understand the roles and responsibilities of specialists in Canada.
   - Understand the organizations and functions of the Canadian healthcare system.
   - Understand the forces of change.
   - Work effectively within teams of colleagues.
   - Manage a medical practice while simultaneously functioning within broader organizational management systems (e.g., hospital committees).
4. *Utilize information technology effectively to optimize patient care, continued self-learning, and other activities.* This includes the ability to do the following:
   - Use patient-related databases.
   - Access computer-based information.
   - Understand the fundamentals of medical informatics.

The Role of Health Advocate

A health advocate responds to challenges represented by those social, environmental, and biological factors that determine the health of patients and society. Advocacy is an essential and fundamental component of health promotion that occurs at the level of the individual patient, the practice population, and the broader community. As a health advocate, a specialist responds both individually and collectively in influencing public health and policy. As delineated in the *CanMEDS 2000 Project Report*, as a health advocate, a specialist should be able to demonstrate the following competencies:

1. *Identify the determinants of health that affect patients in order to be able to effectively contribute to improving individual and societal health in Canada.* This includes the ability to do the following:
   - Recognize, assess, and respond to the psychosocial, economic, and biologic factors influencing the health of those served.
   - Incorporate information on health determinants into personal practice behaviors, both with individual patients and their communities.
   - Adapt patient management and education to promote health, enhance understanding, foster coping abilities, and enhance active participation in informed decision-making.
2. *Recognize and respond to those issues, settings, circumstances, or situations in which advocacy on behalf of patients, professions, or society as appropriate.* This includes the ability to do the following:
   - Identify populations at risk.
   - Identify current policies that affect health.
   - Recognize the fundamental role of epidemiological research in informing practice.

- Describe how public policy is developed.
- Employ methods of influencing the development of health and social policy.

The Role of Scholar

In the role of scholar, a specialist engages in the lifelong pursuit of professional expertise. Recognizing the need to learn continually, the specialist models lifelong learning for others. As a scholar, the specialist contributes to the appraisal, collection, and understanding of healthcare knowledge and facilitates the education of students, patients, and others. As delineated in the *CanMEDS 2000 Project Report*, as a scholar, a specialist should be able to demonstrate the following competencies:

1. *Develop, implement, and document a personal continuing education strategy.* This includes the ability to do the following:
   - Accept responsibility for personal learning needs.
     - Assess personal learning needs.
     - Select appropriate learning methods and materials.
     - Evaluate the outcome of learning to optimize practice.
2. *Apply the principles of critical appraisal to sources of medical information.* This includes the ability to do the following:
   - Incorporate a spirit of scientific inquiry and use of evidence into clinical decision-making.
     - Select appropriate inquiry questions.
     - Efficiently search for and assess the quality of evidence in literature.
     - Keep up-to-date with the evidence-based standard of care for the conditions most commonly seen in patients
3. *Serve as an educator by facilitating the learning of patients, students, residents, and other health professionals.* This includes the ability to do the following:
   - Help others define learning needs and directions for development.
   - Provide constructive feedback to peers and other learners.
   - Apply the principles of adult learning in interactions with patients, students, residents, colleagues, and others.
4. *Contribute to the development of new knowledge.* This includes the ability to do the following:
   - Possess the skills necessary to participate in collaborative research projects, quality assurance, or guideline development relevant to the practice of a specialist.

The Role of Professional

Medical specialists have unique societal roles as professionals with a distinct body of knowledge, skills, and attitudes relevant to improving the health and well-being of others. In the role of professional, the specialist is committed to the highest standards of excellence in clinical care and ethical conduct, continually perfecting mastery of the given medical specialty. As delineated in the *CanMEDS 2000 Project Report*, as a professional, a specialist should be able to demonstrate the following competencies:

1. *Deliver the highest quality care with integrity, honesty, and compassion.* This includes the ability to do the following:
   - Demonstrate an awareness of racial, cultural, and societal issues that impact the delivery of care to patients.
   - Demonstrate an ability to maintain and enhance appropriate knowledge, skills, and professional behaviors.
2. *Exhibit appropriate personal and interpersonal professional behaviors.* This includes the ability to do the following:
   - Assume responsibility for personal actions.
   - Demonstrate a high degree of self-awareness.
   - Maintain an appropriate balance between personal and professional roles.
   - Address interpersonal differences in professional relations.
3. *Practice medicine in an ethically responsible manner that respects the medical, legal, and professional obligations of belonging to a self-regulating body.* This includes the ability to do the following:
   - Demonstrate an understanding of and adherence to legal and ethical codes of practice.
   - Recognize ethical dilemmas and the need to help resolve them.
   - Demonstrate the ability to recognize and respond to unprofessional behaviors in clinical practice, taking into account local and provincial regulations.

IMPLEMENTING THE ROLE FRAMEWORK

Besides delineating the roles a competent specialist must play, the Royal College has and continues to develop tools to implement the roles framework. These tools are meant to assist in learning, teaching, evaluating, and developing faculty. A delineation of these tools as listed in the *CanMEDS 2000 Project Report* is found in Table 3.2.

DIRECTIONS FOR FACULTY DEVELOPMENT

The *CanMEDS 2000 Project Report* stresses that the success of any educational program is greatly influenced by the effectiveness of the faculty. They must have the knowledge, skills, and attitudes appropriate to their medical specialty in addition to the knowledge, skills, and attitudes to design, implement, and evaluate a course of study. They must also be able to evaluate their students' learning and their own effectiveness as teachers. Within the scholar role, the *CanMEDS 2000 Project Report*

Table 3.2 Overview of Educational Strategies for Implementation of Roles

Roles	Learning Environment	Bedside Teaching	Structure: Cognitive Instruction (e.g., case discussions, half-day rounds)	Workshops
Medical Expert	Self-directed learning Individual mentorship	Apprenticeship model	Problem-based learning Clinical reasoning	Effective consultations Presentation skills Evidence-based medicine Information access/retrieval Bioethics
Communicator	Empathy, respect (reflects how patient is treated) Individual and group Reflection of experiences	Role modeling Effective patient and family communications	Conceptual framework of patient-MD communication Communication skills, special topics (e.g., racial/cultural issues, bad news)	Communication skills Constructive feedback Role playing, +/- videotape
Collaborator	Interdisciplinary organization/staffing Seamless healthcare delivery unit (inpatient/ambulatory)	Role modeling	Relevant governance structures Interdisciplinary teaching sessions	Team-building exercises

Role				
Manager	Role modeling, managing time & resources among different priorities		Allocation of healthcare resources	Practice management Leadership skills
Health Advocate	Individual patient and patient population advocacy issues		Relevant governance structures Interdisciplinary teaching sessions	Effective intervention/assistance in patient and population problems
Scholar	Self-directed learning Evidence-based practice Life long learning Practice reflection	Learning from clinical problems	Clinical standard setting Quality assurance/ Management Health economics	Reflection on practice Critical appraisal skills
Professional	Direct observation and feedback Learner prescriptions	Role modeling of professional attitudes and behaviors	Case-based discussions Medico-legal rounds Medical ethics rounds	Awareness of professional responsiblities

discusses functioning as an educator in facilitating learning. Such a role is multi-dimensional as the physician as educator will likely need to function as teacher, professional within the subject area field, researcher, educational design specialist, communicator, performer, coach, advocate, mentor, judge, and remediator. The *CanMEDS 2000 Project Report* clearly points out that faculty development is extremely important in the process of curriculum change. It is all the more important in a project such as *CanMEDS 2000* given that professional attitudes, behaviors, and patterns of practice are more firmly established during postgraduate training than at any other time in the medical life cycle.

The Royal College emphasizes that our commitment to faculty development is not only structured and long-term, but it also places faculty development within the lifelong learning plans of the faculty themselves.

Just as the role of medical expert was central among all the roles a specialist must play, so is the role of mentor central among all of the roles a physician educator must play. As the *CanMEDS Project Report* points out, students implicitly model themselves after their mentors, incorporating in themselves similar concepts, approaches, and attitudes, as well as specific knowledge and skills. It is often through the implicit influences of such role models that students determine their values, priorities, and behaviors. Faculty must not only be knowledgeable about the CanMEDS roles framework of competencies, but they must also exemplify the very behaviors that need to be instilled in students and actively support and promote their application.

Our *CanMEDS 2000 Project Report* also stresses the support that the faculty must have in order to do their task. Faculty require the sustained leadership of senior staff, fair and consistent evaluation, and appropriate career advancement, including financial rewards. The faculty must see the faculty development program as an integral part of their own continuing education programs.

IMPLICATIONS OF THE *CanMEDS 2000 PROJECT* FOR AMERICAN MEDICAL SYSTEMS

Size and Scope

The Royal College is an organization of medical specialists dedicated to ensuring the highest standards and quality of healthcare. Our College is uniquely structured to cover the full spectrum of postgraduate medical education for all fifty-eight medical, surgical, and laboratory specialties recognized in Canada. In other words, the Royal College combines the functions of the Accreditation Council for Graduate Medical Education (ACGME) (with its oversight for the residency programs and the Residency Review Councils) and the American Board of Medical Specialties (ABMS) (with its coordination of medical specialty Boards) within a single organization. Having one organization that is totally responsible for medical specialties allows the implementation of a program of competencies a unified approach. The Royal College is the Canadian institution responsible for all standard setting and monitoring of specialty medical education; the College does this by using specialty-specific committees. To achieve agreement on a body of core competencies and to fully implement them, medical institutions in the United States, would require both the consensus and the complicity of various organizations – a task that could be both time-consuming and tedious, if not absolutely impossible. Our Canadian system is far more streamlined than that which exists in the United States.

Also, all Royal College accredited programs are university-sponsored. There are sixteen medical schools in Canada with university-based programs, sixteen psychiatry residencies, and fifteen neurology residencies. This again contrasts greatly with the United States, which has 125 medical schools, which are sponsored both publicly and privately. In addition, in the United States, there are 179 psychiatry residencies and 117 neurology residencies. The size, scope, and varying governing bodies of the United States' institutions again provide a challenge for the uniform implementation of even the very best programs.

Implementation Procedures

Once the generic competencies were identified, the Royal College embarked on a period of experimentation and development of the CanMEDS roles. This was done through the provision of seed grants to working groups with the overall goal of developing pilot projects on how to teach and evaluate the CanMEDS.

The next phase of implementation for the *CanMEDS 2000 Project* was to incorporate the CanMEDS competencies into the standards and infrastructure of the Royal College. Research and development grants were created, and an Educational Research and Development Unit of the Office of Education was formed. Following that, the CanMEDS competencies were incorporated into the specialty-specific objectives of training, examination blueprints, final in-training evaluation reports, and standards of accreditation are well underway. The specialty-specific objectives of training define each discipline and state the general as well as the specialty-specific objectives under each CanMEDS competency. A sample of these specialty-specific objectives can be found in Table 3.3.

Similar to the observations in the previous section, the monolithic structure of the Royal College has permitted a uniform implementation plan of the "roles concept" that can reach and affect all areas of medical specialty education while still allowing for the uniqueness of specialty-specific competencies. With the diversity of medical specialty training venues in the United States, such an implementation plan would be impossible.

Evaluation Measures on the Residency Level

A new template has been developed for the Final In-Training (residency) Evaluation Reports (FITER) of all specialties and subspecialties recognized by the Royal College. This FITER template incorporates the competencies from each of the seven CanMEDS physician roles. The template identifies the generic competencies required of all specialists, and each Specialty Committee defines specialty-specific competencies as necessary for their FITER.

Table 3.3 Objectives of Training for Neurology Under the Health Advocate Role

General Requirements

- Identify the important determinants of health affecting patients
- Contribute effectively to improved health of patients and communities
- Recognize and respond to those issues where advocacy is appropriate

Specific Requirements

- Learn about community resources and related patient support groups; provide assistance to access programs (e.g., home care, occupational and physiotherapy, drug plans, application for nursing homes, etc.) and participate in their activities
- Educate, be able to generate and access information (e.g., printed material, video-tapes, web sites) and be available as a resource person to counsel patients effectively on neurological disorders
- Counsel patients on the importance of taking responsibility for their own well-being and recognize the important determinants predisposing to neurological disorders (e.g., risk factors for transient ischemic attack (TIA) and stroke, teratogenic effects of anti-epileptic drugs)
- Understand the role of national and international bodies (e.g., Alzheimer, Stroke, Multiple Sclerosis Societies) in the promotion of neurological health, and the prevention, detection, and treatment of neurological disorders

Once each of the disciplines has incorporated its specialty-specific objectives into the FITER, a successful FITER becomes one of the requirements for eligibility to sit for the examinations leading to certification as well as for successful completion of subspecialties without examination. A FITER template using the Medical Expert Role is provided as an example (Table 3.4).

The Canadian FITER template could prove useful to medical residency programs in the United States as a model for a means of evaluating residents on the agreed upon competencies for a given specialty. Given that the medical competencies for each specialty are in the process of being defined, it is possible that the Residency Review Committees could have the responsibility for developing a FITER-like tool to assess residents. A program director's attestation of the completion of a FITER, in combination with other criteria, could serve as a final tool to be required for eligibility for the certification examination.

Examination Blueprints

The Canadian system provides for the initial certification of medical specialists, stressing a comprehensive examination at the end of the training period. The Royal College examination blueprints are based on the CanMEDS competencies as well as on the objectives of training developed by each specialty. An examination blueprint defines the content and competencies that are to be measured by examination.

Table 3.4   FITER Template Using the Medical Expert Role

A rationale must be provided to support ratings with asterisks.	EXPECTATIONS				
	*Rarely meets	*Inconsistently	Generally	Sometimes	*Consistently
MEDICAL EXPERT					
a) Demonstrates a good understanding of the basic scientific and clinical knowledge relevant to the specialty.					
b) History and physical examinations are complete, accurate and well organized.					
c) Uses all of the pertinent information to arrive at complete and accurate clinical decisions.					
d) Recognizes and manages emergency conditions (extremely ill patient) resulting in prompt and appropriate treatment. Remains calm, acts in a timely manner and prioritizes correctly.					
Please define other competencies as necessary.					
Please comment on the strengths and weaknesses of the candidate and provide a rationale for your ratings.					

Blueprints promote content validity (the concept that the examination is designed to test the material it should test), ensure stability of test content and competencies over time, and help in examining the relationship between examination components. Blueprints are used to choose the appropriate measurement technique to evaluate each competency and to weigh the value of the examination components, content, and competencies.

Sample examination blueprints for the general roles of health advocate and scholar are provided in Table 3.5. The examination methodologies listed below include multiple-choice questions, short answer questions, oral examinations, and a composite evaluation of the phenomenology, diagnosis, and management of the competency. In the last-mentioned methodology, technical skills are both tabulated and rated. For those competencies for which none of the cited evaluation methodologies would be appropriate, other evaluative measures must be determined.

The above template may prove useful to the medical specialty boards in the United States if the six categories of core competencies comprise the first column,

Table 3.5 Competencies Table

Roles	Competencies	MCQ	SAQ	ORAL	PDM
Health Advocate	Ability to engage in advocacy activities in responding to the challenges represented by social, environmental, and biological factors				
	Ability to recognize advocacy concept as it relates to the individual patient, the practice population, and the broader community	Y	Y		Y
	Awareness of the major regional, national and international advocacy groups active in mental health matters	Y	Y		
Scholar	Ability, motivation and desire to maintain competence through involvement in independent learning and continuing medical education activities				
	Ability to access and critically appraise sources of medical information	Y	Y		Y
	Ability to facilitate learning of patients, students, residents and other health professionals				Y
	Skills necessary to participate in collaborative research projects quality management, or guidelines development relevant to the practice				

For rows in which no assessment listed is appropriate (i.e., rows where "Y" does not appear) a different type of assessment strategy must be sought.

a listing of all of the competencies comprises the second column, and rather than the evaluation methodologies being listed as above, the sections of the certification and recertification examinations could be listed. Perhaps this listing for certification examinations given by the ABPN could include the Part I (written) examinations and each of the components of the Part II (oral) examination (e.g., patient examination, videotapes, vignettes) as appropriate.

SUMMARY

The CanMEDS Program represents one way of approaching using competencies for training and evaluation purposes. The fact that Canada's core competencies are broken out by the roles that a physician plays as opposed to categories of skills, and the fact that Canada's medical system is structured very differently from that of the United States are irrelevant. The Canadian experience is similar enough in purpose to the core competency movement within the United States that perhaps a great deal of the competency work we have already struggled through can be helpful to our southern neighbors.

NOTES

1. Copies of this report are available from the Royal College of Physicians and Surgeons of Canada, through the Educational Research and Development Unit of the Office of Education, 774 Echo Drive, Ottawa, Ontario, Canada K1S 5N8, telephone 1-800-668-3740/613-730-6276. The report is also available on the Royal College Web Site: http://rcspc.medical.org; refer to Publications and Documents, Special Projects and Reports.

2. In addition, the Royal College Office of Education is responsible for recognition of specialties, accreditation of residency programs, credentialing of candidates, all specialty examinations, and educational research and faculty development. Currently the Royal College recognizes fifty-eight specialties and subspecialties. Each discipline has its own Royal College Specialty Committee. The role of a Specialty Committee is to develop specialty-specific objectives of training and specialty training requirements, develop and update the specific standards of accreditation and is involved in all matters relating to the discipline including review of accreditation status of programs and specialty-specific training requirements.

REFERENCES

Skills for the New Millennium: Report of the Societal Needs Working Group *CanMEDS 2000 Project Report*. The Royal College of Physicians and Surgeons of Canada, 1996

4

The ACGME and ABMS Initiatives Toward the Development of Core Competencies

Susan E. Adamowski, Ed.D.

THE PUSH FOR DEFINITION OF MEDICAL COMPETENCIES

The field of education was heavily influenced during the late 1960s and early 1970s by a focus on educational outcomes. According to Ralph Tyler, a professor at the University of Chicago, educational activities should be guided by objectives written in behavioral terms that describe measurable outcomes. The success of the educational activities should be judged on how well the students achieve the measurable outcomes (Tyler 1949). The concept of core competencies grew out of this focus on educational outcomes and received a major thrust in the 1980s when the U.S. Department of Education mandated outcome measures for all educational projects, including those involving accreditation.

Heavily funded medical education systems, having expanded greatly during the 1970s, were a prime target of this initiative and were called upon to provide evidence of responsible stewardship in preparing competent physicians to meet public healthcare needs. Various groups, meeting through the 1990s, developed objectives to assess or measure these educational outcomes within medicine. Some groups concentrated on attributes of competence, while others focused more on performance issues. These outcomes eventually came to be referred to as necessary, or "core," competencies. Among the groups in the United States working on definitions or delineations of competence were the following:

- The American Board of Medical Specialties (ABMS) Task Force on Competence
- The Accreditation Council for Graduate Medical Education (ACGME) Outcome Project Advisory Group
- The Association of American Medical Colleges' Medical School Objectives Project Group

- The Federated Council for Internal Medicine Task Force on the Internal Medicine Residency Curriculum
- The National Association for Competency Assurance
- The Pew Health Professions Commission

The work of these various groups was remarkably similar. The Core Components of Competence as listed by the ABMS in draft form for discussion at its March 16–17, 1999 Task Force on Competence Meeting is provided in Table 4.1.

Table 4.1 ABMS Example Components of Competence (see Note 1)

Attributes	Example Components
Medical Knowledge	• Possess up-to-date knowledge needed to evaluate and manage patients
Clinical Skills	• Demonstrate proficiency in history-taking • Conduct physical examinations effectively • Lead and manage diagnostic studies • Demonstrate practice skills • Show proficiency in technical skills
Clinical Judgment	• Demonstrate clinical reasoning • Make sound diagnostic and therapeutic decisions • Understand the limits of one's knowledge • Incorporate the considerations of cost-awareness and risk-benefit analysis for the patient
Interpersonal Skills	• Communicate and work effectively with patients, families, physicians, other health professionals, and health-related agencies
Professional Attitudes and Behavior	*Accountability* • Accept responsibility • Maintain comprehensive, timely, and legible medical records • Be available in a consultative role to other physicians and health professionals when needed • Seek continuous improvement in the quality of care provided • Facilitate learning of patients, students, housestaff, and other health professionals. *Lifelong Learning* • Evaluate critically new medical and scientific information relevant to the practice of medicine and apply it to patient care • Possess skills and experience in self-assessment of medical knowledge and clinical skills

(*continued*)

Table 4.1   ABMS Example Components of Competence (see Note 1)—cont'd

Attributes	Example Components
	Humanistic Qualities • Demonstrate integrity and honesty • Demonstrate compassion/empathy • Show respect for patients' privacy • Show respect for the dignity of patients as persons, including their culture, gender, and age
	Ethical Behavior • Consistently demonstrate high standards of moral and ethical behavior
Managerial Skills	• Work effectively and efficiently in a healthcare organization • Utilize information technology to optimize patient care, lifelong learning, and other activities • Possess basic business skills important for effective practice management
Health Advocacy	• Promote health and prevention of disease of individuals and populations • Advocate in the interest of one's patients

Essentially at the same time as the above list was being discussed by the ABMS, the ACGME asked its Outcome Project Advisory Group to research work on competencies and to develop a list of necessary competencies. The group eventually settled on 86 competencies for physicians, and that list was pared to six general areas:

- Patient Care
- Medical Knowledge (originally Clinical Science)
- Interpersonal and Communications Skills
- Practice-Based Learning and Improvement
- Professionalism
- Systems-Based Practice

Within these six major categories, the ACGME's Outcome Project Advisory Group listed competencies in a manner similar to the way the ABMS had listed the components of its necessary attributes of competency as shown in Table 4.1. A major step forward occurred in September 1999 when the ABMS Assembly agreed to adopt the ACGME's six areas of competencies. This meant that for the first time there was agreement on the areas of core competencies among the governing body of residency programs and the umbrella organization over medical specialty boards.

The chart provided here (Table 4.2) lists the competencies with the six categories as written by the ACGME and correlates those with the ABMS components

Table 4.2 General Competencies Core Components (see Note 2)

Categories	ACGME	ABMS	CanMEDS 2000 Project
Patient Care	Communicate effectively and demonstrate caring and respectful behaviors when interacting with patients	Demonstrate proficiency in history-taking	Medical Expert
			Communicator
		Conduct physical examinations effectively	
	Gather essential and accurate information about the patient and use it together with up-to-date scientific evidence to make decisions about diagnostic and therapeutic interventions	Lead and manage diagnostic studies	
		Demonstrate clinical reasoning	
		Understand the limits of one's knowledge	
	Develop and carry out patient management plans	Make sound diagnostic and therapeutic decisions	
	Perform competently all medical and invasive procedures considered essential for the area of practice	Demonstrate practice skills	
		Show proficiency in technical skills	
	Provide healthcare services aimed at preventing health problems or maintaining health	Promote health and prevention of disease of individuals and populations	

Category	Competency		Role
	Work with other healthcare professionals to provide patient-focused care that maximizes the likelihood of a positive health outcome	Advocate in the interest of one's patients	
		Utilize information technology to optimize patient care, lifelong learning, and other activities	Medical Expert
Medical Knowledge (Clinical Science)	Demonstrate rigor in thinking about clinical situations	Possess up-to-date knowledge needed to evaluate and manage patients	
	Know and apply the basic and clinically supportive sciences which are appropriate to the discipline		
Practice-Based Learning and Improvement	Analyze practice experience and perform practice-based improvement activities using a systematic methodology	Evaluate critically new medical and scientific information relevant to the practice of medicine and apply it to patient care	Scholar
	Locate, appraise, and assimilate "best practices" related to patients' health problems	Utilize information technology to optimize patient care, lifelong learning, and other activities	Manager
	Apply knowledge of study designs and statistical methods to the appraisal of clinical studies and other information on diagnostic and therapeutic effectiveness	Possess skills and experience in self-assessment of medical knowledge and clinical skills	

(continued)

Table 4.2 General Competencies Core Components (see Note 2)—cont'd

Categories	ACGME	ABMS	CanMEDS 2000 Project
	Use the computer to manage information, access on-line medical information, and support clinical care and patient education	Facilitate learning of patients, students, housestaff, and other health professionals	
Interpersonal and Communications Skills	Create and sustain a therapeutic relationship with patients	Communicate and work effectively with patients, families, physicians, other health professionals, and health-related agencies	Communicator
	Engage in active listening, provide information using appropriate language, ask clear questions, and provide an opportunity for input and questions	Be available in a consultative role to other physicians and health professionals when needed	Collaborator
	Work effectively as a member or leader of a healthcare team or other professional group	Maintain comprehensive, timely, and legible medical records	
Professionalism	Demonstrate respect, regard, integrity, and a responsiveness to the needs of patients and society that supercedes self-interest; assume responsibility and act responsibly; demonstrate a commitment to excellence	Accept responsibility	Professional
		Demonstrate integrity and honesty	Scholar/Health Advocate
		Demonstrate compassion/empathy	
		Show respect for patients' privacy	
	Demonstrate a commitment to ethical principles pertaining to provision or withholding of clinical care,	Consistently demonstrate high standards of moral and ethical behavior	

		Health Advocate
	Show respect for the dignity of patients as persons, including their culture, gender, and age	
	confidentiality of patient information, informed consent, and business practices	
	Demonstrate sensitivity and responsiveness to cultural differences, including awareness of one's own and one's patients cultural perspectives	
Systems-Based Practice	Understand how patient care practices and related actions impact component units of the healthcare delivery system and the total delivery system, and how delivery systems impact the provision of healthcare	Incorporate the considerations of cost-awareness and risk-benefit analysis for the patient
		Advocate in the interest of one's patients
	Know systems-based approaches to controlling healthcare costs and allocating resources; practice cost-effective healthcare and resource allocating that does not compromise quality of care	Work effectively and efficiently in a healthcare organization
		Possess basic business skills important for effective practice management
	Advocate for quality patient care and assist patients dealing with system complexities	Seek continuous improvement in the quality of care provided
	Know how to partner with healthcare managers and healthcare providers to assess, coordinate, and improve healthcare; know how these activities can impact system performance	

listed in Table 4.1 and the seven roles a physician plays as delineated by the *CanMEDS Project* of the Royal College of Physicians and Surgeons of Canada as described in Chapter 3.

Concurrent with the implementation of core competencies at the residency level according to ACGME mandate, the ABMS announced that it expected specialty Boards to determine which components of each competency are relevant to their specialty initial certification and maintenance of certification programs. Later, in March 2002, the ABMS Assembly approved, as part of Maintenance of Certification©, "Guidelines for the Assessment of Physician Practice performance." The guidelines stated that initially, each of the six general competencies should be assessed at least once during a Board's repeating Maintenance of Certification cycle.

To complete these tasks, quadrads composed of a specialty Board representative, an ACGME Residency Review Committee (RRC) representative, a program director, and a resident, were established through the Joint Initiative of the ACGME Outcome Project and the ABMS. The quadrads each developed a specialty-specific version and an assessment plan for each of the competencies. The neurology Quadrad members were Dr. Nicholas A. Vick representing the American Board of Psychiatry and Neurology (ABPN); Dr. Rosalie Burns representing the Neurology RRC; Dr. Wendy Peltier, the neurology program director at the Medical College of Wisconsin; and Dr. Shannon Kilgore, representing neurology residents.

THE PRODUCT OF THE QUADRAD IN NEUROLOGY

The outline of the six general categories of core competencies as developed by the Neurology Quadrad can be found in the Appendix.

A COMPARISON OF THE QUADRAD OUTLINES

The quadrads for the different medical specialties came up with a variety of approaches to their outline task. All quadrad outlines, however, were set up in essentially the same way, as they had to relate to the six areas of core competencies as agreed upon by the ACGME and the ABMS.

The difference between the neurology and psychiatry quadrad outlines became a cause for concern for the ABPN, since the Board is unique in representing two specialties. The history of this merger goes back to the inception of the ABPN in 1934. Because the ABPN represents two specialties, the Task Force on Core Competencies, the body established by the ABPN to consider the ACGME/ABMS mandate regarding core competencies, suggested that the two quadrad outlines be merged so that the ABPN would have one core competency outline for which to be responsible to the ABMS.

Generally speaking, the Psychiatry Quadrad Outline was more specific than the Neurology Quadrad Outline. In addition, the Psychiatry Quadrad Outline offered suggestions for evaluative tools at the end of each outline section. The Neurology Quadrad included its evaluation suggestions in a table attached to the end of its outline.

While the approaches to content in the various sections of the outline required discussion, the discrepancy between the two Medical Knowledge sections was the most dichotomous. The Neurology Quadrad basically said through their outline that neurology residents must be competent in two areas:

1. Neurology residents must know the areas of medical knowledge as provided in the content outlines of the examinations given by the ABPN. (Note: This section of the Neurology Quadrad Outline attaches the content outline for the ABPN written certification [Part I] examination in neurology.)

2. Neurology residents must have the ability to reference and utilize electronic information systems to access new information.

The Neurology Quadrad's attaching the ABPN examination content outline as essentially their complete Medical Knowledge section of the core competencies outline raised an interesting question: Should the Medical Knowledge section of the core competency outline be exactly the same as the Board's examination content outline in that specialty? The Neurology Quadrad thought that it should, but the Psychiatry Quadrad differed and wrote its own list of core competencies for the Medical Knowledge category. An examination of other specialty quadrad outlines shows that a variety of approaches was taken in this and other areas.

In dealing with the six different subject areas of the core competencies outline (Patient Care, Medical Knowledge, Interpersonal and Communications Skills, Practice-Based Learning and Improvement, Professionalism, and Systems-Based Practice), a dichotomy emerged. It appeared that while the first two content sections of the outline (Patient Care and Medical Knowledge) were divergent, the content of the last four sections of the outline (Interpersonal and Communications Skills, Practice-Based Learning and Improvement, Professionalism, and Systems-Based Practice) was more similar than divergent. Thus, it appeared that the latter four sections of the outline would be easier to merge than the first two.

Reflection suggested the logic behind this observation. Physicians' skills in the last four areas of the outline (Interpersonal and Communications Skills, Practice-Based Learning and Improvement, Professionalism, and Systems-Based Practice) could be thought of as being more uniform across specialties than specific to a specialty. The first two areas of the outline (Patient Care and Medical Knowledge) would be, logically, more specialty-specific. To deal with this dichotomy, it was decided to merge the first two sections of the neurology competency outline with the psychiatry competency outline as far as possible. These common areas would be referred to as "General Patient Care" and "General Medical Knowledge." The specialty-specific areas of Patient Care and Medical

Knowledge would be kept separate and labeled "Neurology" and "Psychiatry" as appropriate.

It was further decided that the last four sections of the competency outlines would be merged into one with a uniform format. Rather than use the statements/bulleted points format of the neurology outline or the numbered statements/bulleted points of the psychiatry outline, a regular "Roman numeral" outline format was selected for this merger.

THE MERGED CORE COMPETENCY OUTLINE

Through the process of merging the Psychiatry Quadrad outline and the Neurology Quadrad outline, it became abundantly clear that core competencies, in concept, are fluid and responsive to new knowledge in the medical field and to advances in technology among other things. Thus, the task of arriving at a "final" core competency outline was once and for all time abandoned. Any iteration of a core competency outline can only be current as of its writing. Amendments and revisions will always need to be made, and all those who use the core competency outlines (e.g., medical school faculty, program residency directors, medical certification examination writers) will need to take this principle into account. Clear communication among core competency constituent groups regarding major changes in the core competencies outline would be absolutely necessary, but most variations would be assumed to be minor.

A "final version" of the core competency outline was prepared after having taken into account input from all of the ABPN directors. This "final version" of the core competency outline was final only in the sense that it was the outline that was printed for use at the ABPN Invitational Core Competencies Conference, which is discussed in Section III of this book. Changes to the outline were anticipated and accepted during the work of that conference.

Acknowledgments

The author is indebted to Dr. David Leach, Executive Director of the Accreditation Council for Graduate Medical Education, and Dr. Sheldon D. Horowitz, Associate Vice President of the American Board of Medical Specialties, for their assistance in the preparation of this chapter.

NOTES

1. Adapted from the meeting held in Chicago, IL, American Board of Medical Specialties Task Force on Competence Agenda Book for March 16–17, 1999, pp. 91–92.

2. The first three columns of this chart are from the meeting in Chicago, IL, American Board of Medical Specialties Task Force on Competence Agenda

Book for March 16–17, 1999, pp. 93–96. The fourth column is adapted from the same source, p. 107.

REFERENCES

Tyler RW. Basic Principles of Curriculum and Instruction: Syllabus for Education 360. Chicago. University of Chicago Press, 1949.

Core Competencies and the Practice of Neurology Today: The ABPN Initiative

This section of the book will focus on the key points that emerged from the discussions conducted at the American Board of Psychiatry and Neurology (ABPN) Invitational Core Competencies Conference held June 22–23, 2001 in Toronto, Ontario, Canada. For this conference, the ABPN invited some of the key leaders in the medical fields of neurology and psychiatry to come together to discuss the six categories of core competencies as agreed upon by the Accreditation Council on Graduate Medical Education (ACGME) and the American Board of Medical Specialties (ABMS). Approximately fifty of the invitees were able to attend. The primary goal of the conference was for the thought leaders in medical education to dialogue about how best to implement the core competencies as written for certification purposes.

Representatives from the following groups were initially invited to the ABPN Core Competencies Conference:

- Accreditation Council for Continuing Medical Education
- Accreditation Council for Graduate Medical Education
- American Academy of Child and Adolescent Psychiatry
- American Academy of Neurology
- American Association of Chairpersons of Departments of Psychiatry
- American Association of Directors of Psychiatric Residency Training
- American Association of Medical Colleges
- American Board of Medical Specialties
- American College of Psychiatrists
- American Medical Association
- American Neurological Association
- American Psychiatric Association
- Association of University Professors of Neurology
- Child Neurology Society
- National Institute of Mental Health
- National Institute of Neurological Disorders and Stroke

- Professors of Child Neurology
- Royal College of Physicians and Surgeons of Canada
- Substance Abuse and Mental Health Services Administration

Working objectives presented for the ABPN Invitational Core Competencies Conference were as follows:

1. Determine what core competencies for neurology and psychiatry should be assessed for certification purposes.
2. Determine who should do the assessment. (If not ABPN, then who?)
3. Determine how this should be done. (Which assessment methodologies should be used for which competencies?)
4. Determine where in the medical education track this should be done. (If by ABPN, at which assessment?)
5. Determine how to collect data to validate the core competencies.

In addition to the questions in the objectives above, two other key issues needed attention. These were the following:

1. Is the core competency outline as currently conceived adequate for ABPN purposes? If not, what needs to be changed, and how?
2. Are there core competencies about psychiatry that neurologists need to know (and vice versa) to be judged competent? If so, what must be added to the outline?

Nadia Z. Mikhael, M.D., Director of Education for the Royal College of Physicians and Surgeons of Canada, delivered a keynote address to the conference participants. Her topic was the pioneering work done by the Royal College regarding core competencies. Specifically, Dr. Mikhael focused on the following:

1. Listing the competencies that the *CanMEDS 2000 Project* identified as being needed by physician specialists.
2. Explaining how the Royal College went about working with program directors and curriculum committees to assure that the necessary material covering these competencies was taught in residency.

Dr. Mikhael's presentation at the conference is the basis for her chapter in the preceding section (Section II, Chapter 3).

The chapters in Section III present in some detail the discussions that occurred as breakout groups of conference participants attempted to accomplish the tasks set by the conference objectives. Each breakout group was assigned to one of the six general areas of core competencies. Discussion was structured by applying the objectives to each individual competency within each of the six general core competency areas. While the discussion groups did come to some specific conclusions, discussion tended to be global rather than specific. Chapters 5 through 10 discuss each of the core competency areas as it applies to the field of neurology. Chapter 11 discusses which psychiatry competencies are necessary for neurologists to know.

Following the small group work, the group reconvened as a large group for reports on the general core competency areas. Questions and answers followed each small group presentation. The conference concluded with remarks from a selected panel of reactors. The remarks included subjective evaluations of the conference and various answers to the unspoken question, "Where do we go from here with the core competencies?" Section IV of this book will discuss these issues.

5

General and Neurology-Specific Patient Care Core Competencies

Nicholas A. Vick, M.D.

ASSUMPTIONS REGARDING THE PATIENT CARE CORE COMPETENCIES

The group discussing the Patient Care Core Competency section of the outline debated several initial assumptions. First, they assumed that every competency listed for them to consider was already being assessed by the American Board of Psychiatry and Neurology (ABPN) written certification (Part I) examination, by the ABPN oral certification (Part II) examination, or by both. Second, they also assumed that the Patient Care Core Competencies should all be of the highest priority for both training and assessment purposes. Both of these assumptions were supported after debate, but much discussion ensued regarding the first assumption.

The Patient Care Core Competencies outline is divided into three sections: general, neurology, and psychiatry. The competencies in the general section apply to both neurologists and psychiatrists, but the latter two sections are specialty-specific. For the purposes of this book, the psychiatry section will not be discussed here, but will be referenced in a discussion of cross-competencies in Chapter 11.

The outline as presented to the conference participants was divided into parts, with each part representing essentially one core competency. This division into parts was made by the staff in order to create logical sections of the outline for discussion purposes. It was recognized that the discussion group might want to make changes if they deemed them necessary. This information was communicated to the discussion group leaders in their training, but no changes for the Patient Care Core Competencies were thought to be necessary; thus, each section of the outline discussed below will be assumed, for current purposes, to be one core competency.

DISCUSSION OF THE FIRST GENERAL PATIENT CARE CORE COMPETENCY

The first general Patient Care Core Competency is as follows:

1. *The physician shall demonstrate the ability to perform and document a comprehensive history and examination to include as appropriate:*
   A. Chief complaint
   B. History of present illness
   C. Past medical history
   D. Review of systems
   E. Family history
   F. Social history
   G. Developmental history (especially for children)

The discussants clearly saw this core competency as being assessed primarily through clinical examinations, such as the current ABPN oral certification (Part II) examination. Discussion centered on the difficulty that some candidates have with this examination. Indeed, the demonstration of this competency (and some of the following related core competencies) has proven to be such a stumbling block that some candidates have been unable to pass the patient portion of the Part II examination in spite of multiple attempts.

Discussion led to the idea that if this core competency is such a basic skill, it should be formally assessed early in candidates' educational careers. That way, if remediation were needed, it could be provided while the candidates were still in training. If remediation proved ineffective, then a candidate could be redirected in terms of career decisions. How this assessment task could be accomplished led to more discussion, with one conclusion being that the residency program directors could be the primary assessors of this core competency. The ABPN could work in some manner with the program directors to make certain that the assessment was done according to the Board's current standard.

Further discussion included the necessity for including this core competency in the Practice Assessment Component of the ABPN Maintenance of Certification (MOC) Program. The ABPN MOC Program will affect all practicing neurologists who do not have lifetime certification, that is, those who were certified after October 1, 1994. Neurologists holding lifetime certification will also be able to apply for the ABPN MOC Program to demonstrate their continued competence in practice.

As the ABPN MOC Program is just beginning to be implemented according to the mandate of the American Board of Medical Specialties (ABMS), the discussion directions provided to the group encouraged them to think about using the four components of the MOC Program (Licensure, Self-Assessment and Lifelong Learning, the Recertification Examination, and Practice Assessment) as assessment opportunities for core competencies when appropriate for recertification purposes. Conference participants were told that they need not be concerned at this time as to how the Lifelong Learning and Practice Assessment Components of the ABPN MOC Program were going to be implemented. Decisions regarding these two components of the MOC Program would be made later by the ABPN, most likely with direction from the ABMS. The main issue for discussion at this conference was to see what core competencies might be delegated to the ABPN MOC Program.

Thus, for this first Patient Care Core Competency, the group recorded that this competency is being assessed on the ABPN oral certification (Part II) examination, but that this competency should at least initially be assessed much earlier in the candidates' careers. Program directors, with involvement at some level by the ABPN, could carry out this assessment, and their evaluation would be sufficient for the early part of the candidates' careers. Program directors would also have the responsibility to provide remediation for candidates who did not perform up to standard on this measure of competence. This core competency was also assigned to the Practice Assessment Component of the ABPN MOC Program for neurologists seeking recertification.

Possible methodologies suggested for assessing this core competency included the following:

- Oral examinations with actual patients, similar to what is currently being done in the ABPN oral certification (Part II) examination.
- Oral examinations using standardized patients.
- Vignettes, which could be presented at various points during the candidates' educational journey.
- Objective-structured clinical examinations (OSCEs).

Some conference participants spoke of program directors having a conflict of interest in trying to assess the competence of their own residents. Program directors, because of their involvement with their residents and their need for their program to be seen in a good light, might not be able to rate their residents objectively. It was concluded that the program directors could provide initial assessment in this area, but that someone outside the training program would need to certify that a physician had a particular skill. The assessment provided by the program directors would be especially helpful for those residents needing remediation, as such could easily be provided during residency. There was no consensus as to when this competency should be assessed for certification purposes.

To validate that this core competency is indeed a required competency for the practice of neurology, the perceptions of both public and professional groups could be referenced and documented. Given that, patients could represent the public sector and report their perceptions of encounters with the physicians. While patients could not judge the clinical effectiveness of a physician's work involved with this competency, they could report whether or not different portions of the examination had, in fact, been done. In most cases, during a patient/physician encounter, no one else is present. Thus, the patient is in a unique position to assess the completeness of the tasks listed within the first core competency. Perceptions of other professionals (general physicians, other specialists, and nurses, for example) as to how well the physician accomplishes this core competency would also be important. These could be measured on the basis of feedback given to a referring physician, information provided to a nurse, and discussion about the patient with other specialist colleagues in neurology and/or in other fields.

DISCUSSION OF THE SECOND GENERAL PATIENT CARE CORE COMPETENCY

The second general Patient Care Core Competency is as follows:

2. *The physician shall demonstrate the ability to create differential diagnoses.*

After the extensive discussion of the first Patient Care Core Competency, this second one was handled quickly. Basically, everything that was said regarding the core competency discussed above could also apply to this one. The only addition was that the group thought that this core competency could also be assessed on cognitive examinations, like the ABPN written certification (Part I) examination.

During discussion of all that needed to be assessed on the written and oral sections of the ABPN certification examination, it was pointed out that all examinations, no matter what their form, are *samplings* of representative knowledge, skills, and/or attitudes. No examination can ever test every situation that a professional might encounter in practice.

Therefore, for its written certification (Part I) examination, the ABPN would need to be committed to having a question pool that covered all of the core competencies which could be assessed in a multiple choice question (MCQ) format. Not all questions would have to be asked – or even could be asked – but that is not the goal of an examination. The examination is meant to sample representative knowledge.

Similarly with the ABPN oral certification (Part II) examination, only a sampling of possible patients can be considered. Methods of validation could include both public and professional perception.

DISCUSSION OF THE THIRD GENERAL PATIENT CARE CORE COMPETENCY

The third general Patient Care Core Competency is as follows:

3. *The physician shall demonstrate the ability to evaluate, assess, and recommend cost-effective management of patients.*

Similar to the second general Patient Care Core Competency, for this third core competency, it was assumed that the ABPN written certification (Part I) and oral certification (Part II) examinations, along with the Practice Assessment Component of the MOC Program could be the times this competency would be assessed. Specific suggested methodologies for assessment here included oral interviews, audits, and portfolios. Methods of validation could include outcome studies and both public and professional perception.

DISCUSSION OF THE FIRST NEUROLOGY PATIENT CARE CORE COMPETENCY

The second section of the core competency outline represents neurology-specific core competencies. The first neurology-specific Patient Care Core Competency is as follows:

1. *Based on a comprehensive neurological assessment, the physician shall demonstrate the ability to do the following:*
   A. Determine if a patient's symptoms are the result of a disease affecting the central and/or peripheral nervous system or are of another origin.
   B. Develop and document a formulation, differential diagnosis, laboratory investigation, and management plan.

This core competency was judged to be of the highest priority for assessment purposes. The discussion group believed that it should be assessed on both the ABPN written certification (Part I) and oral certification (Part II) examinations and also as part of the ABPN MOC Program. The discussion group thought that this core competency merited assessment under three of the four components of the MOC Program: through the Lifelong Learning Component, on the Recertification Examination, and through the Practice Assessment Component. For the non-examination portions of this assessment, the group thought that portfolios and supervisor/peer attestations would serve as workable assessment methodologies. Validation of this core competency could be done through both public and professional perceptions as discussed earlier.

DISCUSSION OF THE SECOND NEUROLOGY PATIENT CARE CORE COMPETENCY

The second neurology-specific Patient Care Core Competency is as follows:

2. *Based on a comprehensive neurological assessment, the physician shall demonstrate the technical skills to do the following:*
   A. Perform lumbar puncture, edrophonium, and caloric testing.
   B. Identify and describe abnormalities seen in common neurological disorders on radiographic testing, including plain films, myelography, angiography, computed tomography (CT), isotope, magnetic resonance imaging (MRI), and positron emission tomography (PET)/single photon emission computed tomography (SPECT) imaging of the neuroaxis.

C. Evaluate the application and relevance of investigative procedures and interpretation in the diagnosis of neurological disease, including the following:
1. Electroencephalogram
2. Motor and nerve conduction studies
3. Electromyography
4. Evoked potentials
5. Polysomnography
6. Audiometry
7. Perimetry
8. Psychometry
9. Cerebrospinal fluid (CSF) analysis
10. Vascular imaging (Duplex, transcranial Doppler)
11. Radiographic studies as outlined above
D. Identify and describe gross and microscopic specimens taken from the normal nervous system and from patients with major neurological disorders.

Similar to the first neurology-specific core competency, the discussion group felt this competency, with all its parts, to be of the highest priority for assessment. It was felt that Point A could be assessed only through observation or attestation, which would have to be done by a supervisor. The group felt strongly that this point should be included on the Practice Assessment Component of the ABPN MOC Program.

Also, similar to the first neurology-specific core competency, Points B and C of the second competency could be assessed on the ABPN written certification (Part I) and oral certification (Part II) examinations. Also similar to the first neurology-specific core competency, it was thought that this core competency should be assessed under three parts of the ABPN MOC Program, namely, the Recertification Examination (most likely with multiple choice questions), the Lifelong Learning Component (perhaps with portfolio evaluation), and the Practice Assessment Component.

Program directors could coach their residents on the skills needed to demonstrate this core competency and provide initial assessment feedback. Those candidates needing remediation could receive assistance through their residency programs. This core competency could also be validated using measures of public and professional perceptions.

DISCUSSION OF THE THIRD NEUROLOGY PATIENT CARE CORE COMPETENCY

The third neurology-specific Patient Care Core Competency is as follows:

3. *Based on a comprehensive neurological assessment, the physician shall demonstrate the ability to recognize and treat neurological disorders.*

Like the first neurology-specific core competency and Points B and C of the second neurology-specific core competency, this third core competency was thought to be of utmost importance and assessable under the ABPN written certification (Part I) and oral certification (Part II) examinations and the three previously discussed components of the ABPN MOC Program. This core competency could also be validated using measures of public and professional perceptions.

SUMMARY

The full outline of Patient Care Core Competencies is listed below.

General Patient Care Core Competencies

1. The physician shall demonstrate the ability to perform and document a comprehensive history and examination to include as appropriate:
   A. Chief complaint
   B. History of present illness
   C. Past medical history
   D. Review of systems
   E. Family history
   F. Social history
   G. Developmental history (especially for children)
2. The physician shall demonstrate the ability to create differential diagnoses.
3. The physician shall demonstrate the ability to evaluate, assess, and recommend cost-effective management of patients.

Neurology-Specific Patient Care Core Competencies

1. Based on a comprehensive neurological assessment, the physician shall demonstrate the ability to do the following:
   A. Determine if a patient's symptoms are the result of a disease affecting the central and/or peripheral nervous system or are of another origin.
   B. Develop and document a formulation, differential diagnosis, laboratory investigation, and management plan.
2. Based on a comprehensive neurological assessment, the physician shall demonstrate the technical skills to do the following:
   A. Perform lumbar puncture, edrophonium, and caloric testing.
   B. Identify and describe abnormalities seen in common neurological disorders on radiographic testing, including plain films, myelography, angiography, CT, isotope, MRI, and PET/SPECT imaging of the neuroaxis.
   C. Evaluate the application and relevance of investigative procedures and interpretation in the diagnosis of neurological disease, including the following:
      1. Electroencephalogram
      2. Motor and nerve conduction studies

     3. Electromyography
     4. Evoked potentials
     5. Polysomnography
     6. Audiometry
     7. Perimetry
     8. Psychometry
     9. CSF analysis
    10. Vascular imaging (Duplex, transcranial Doppler)
    11. Radiographic studies as outline above.

  D. Identify and describe gross and microscopic specimens taken from the normal nervous system and from patients with major neurological disorders.

3. Based on a comprehensive neurological assessment, the physician shall demonstrate the ability to recognize and treat neurological disorders.

To summarize, the Patient Care Category of the core competency outline is divided into three sections: a general section; a neurology-specific section; and a psychiatry-specific section. Only the first two sections are discussed here. Psychiatry Patient Care Core Competencies will be covered in Chapter 11, which will deal with what neurologists need to know about psychiatry for their clinical practice.

All of the core competencies in the Patient Care Category of the outline were judged to be of highest priority in terms of assessment. Most of them are currently being assessed by the ABPN written certification (Part I) or oral certification (Part II) examinations, but some topics lend themselves more easily than others to a multiple choice question format. All of the core competencies could be assessed using the ABPN oral certification (Part II) examination, but the competency involving therapeutic skills (the third neurology-specific core competency) could prove both cost- and time-prohibitive.

For all Patient Care Core Competencies, it was agreed that the residency program faculty would be key teachers in assisting residents to master these core competencies. Feedback during the learning process would be important so that remediation, when needed, could occur. Initial assessments by program directors could also serve to hone and perfect skills. It is possible that at some point these core competencies could be assessed during residency, but for certification purposes this would have to be done with the use of an outside evaluator to eliminate conflict of interest issues program directors might have.

Portfolio development, currently in use in some programs to a minor extent, could serve as a possible means of evaluation as long as the focus was on the content of the portfolio and not on its format or façade.

All of the Patient Care Core Competencies could be validated by measurements of perception of the public (singularly represented in each patient) and various professions with which neurologists interact (general physicians, other neurologists, nurses, social workers, etc.).

6

General and Neurology-Specific Medical Knowledge Core Competencies

Harold P. Adams, Jr., M.D.

ASSUMPTIONS REGARDING THE MEDICAL KNOWLEDGE CORE COMPETENCIES

The group discussing the Medical Knowledge Core Competency section of the outline made several initial assumptions, just as the group discussing the Patient Care Core Competencies had done.

- This group's first assumption was that every competency listed for them to consider was already being assessed by cognitive examinations, such as the American Board of Psychiatry and Neurology (ABPN) written certification (Part I) examination, by clinical examinations, such as the ABPN oral certification (Part II) examination, or by both. For the purposes of discussion here, all Medical Knowledge Core Competencies are in fact represented in some way on both the ABPN written examination and oral examination; minor variations from this will be discussed as they arise in the text.
- The group's second assumption was that all of the Medical Knowledge Core Competencies would be of the highest priority for both training and assessment purposes. Minor variations from this general statement will be discussed as they arise in the text.
- The group's third assumption was that all of the Medical Knowledge Core Competencies could be validated as core competencies by using surveys of the field. This assumption proved valid throughout the Medical Knowledge Category of the outline.

DISCUSSION OF THE FIRST GENERAL MEDICAL KNOWLEDGE CORE COMPETENCY

The first general Medical Knowledge Core Competency is as follows:

1. *The physician shall demonstrate knowledge of the major disorders, including the following:*
   A. The epidemiology of the disorder.
   B. The etiology of the disorder, including medical, genetic, and social factors.
   C. The phenomenology of the disorder.
   D. Diagnostic criteria.
   E. Effective treatment strategies.
   F. Course and prognosis.

The discussants clearly saw this core competency as currently being assessed through cognitive examinations, such as the ABPN written certification (Part I) examination, and clinical examinations, such as the current ABPN oral certification (Part II) examination. In addition, the group clearly thought that this competency should be assessed on recertification examinations and possibly also as part of the Practice Assessment Category of the ABPN Maintenance of Certification (MOC) Program.

Methodologies for assessing this competency included in-training evaluations, cognitive examinations, and portfolio assessment. In-training evaluations could take a variety of forms, but would be administered by program directors. The primary goal here would be to identify and assist residents needing remediation. Cognitive examinations would include the multiple choice questions (MCQs) of the ABPN written certification (Part I) examination and recertification examination. Portfolio assessment would most likely be used when actual practice is assessed as part of the ABPN MOC Program.

DISCUSSION OF THE SECOND GENERAL MEDICAL KNOWLEDGE CORE COMPETENCY

The second general Medical Knowledge Core Competency is as follows:

2. *The physician shall demonstrate knowledge of healthcare delivery systems.*

Discussants saw this competency as being evaluated through cognitive and oral examinations and through the Practice Assessment Component of the ABPN MOC Program. Examinations could be part of the training program and/or part of the ABPN certification process. This competency was one of the very few in the Medical Knowledge Category that did not assume a place of first priority among the competencies needing to be assessed. It was ranked, in fact, among the lowest priorities for assessment.

DISCUSSION OF THE THIRD GENERAL MEDICAL KNOWLEDGE CORE COMPETENCY

The third general Medical Knowledge Core Competency is as follows:

3. *The physician shall demonstrate knowledge of ethics in neurology/psychiatry.*

Ethics can be difficult to assess, but the discussion group thought that both cognitive ethical questions could be formulated for MCQ examinations and for clinical testing situations. The group also thought that this competency could be evaluated through the Practice Assessment Component of the ABPN MOC Program. Assessment of this competency could take place in training and/or at the time of certification. It was also thought that state licensing bodies would be involved with the assessment of ethics through their licensure programs.

DISCUSSION OF THE FOURTH GENERAL MEDICAL KNOWLEDGE CORE COMPETENCY

The fourth general Medical Knowledge Core Competency is as follows:

4. *The physician shall demonstrate the ability to reference and utilize electronic information systems to access medical, scientific, and patient information.*

The group believed that this core competency did not warrant assessment at this time, but that this competency should be considered soon for implementation.

DISCUSSION OF THE FIRST NEUROLOGY-SPECIFIC MEDICAL KNOWLEDGE CORE COMPETENCY

The first neurology-specific Medical Knowledge Core Competency is as follows:

1. *The physician shall demonstrate knowledge of basic neuroscience that would be critical to the practice of neurology, including cognitive, behavioral, and social development.*

The discussants felt that this competency could be assessed using MCQs, in-training evaluations, patient interviews, and portfolios. Regarding certification, they saw this competency as being assessed through the ABPN written certification (Part I) and oral certification (Part II) examinations and the recertification examinations. The discussion group judged this competency to be of the highest priority for neurologists.

DISCUSSION OF THE SECOND NEUROLOGY-SPECIFIC MEDICAL KNOWLEDGE CORE COMPETENCY

The second neurology-specific Medical Knowledge Core Competency is as follows:

2. *The physician shall demonstrate knowledge of major neurological and psychiatric disorders and familiarity with the scientific basis of neurological diseases, including the following (see Note 1):*
   A. Neuroanatomy
      1. Cerebral cortex
      2. Connecting systems
      3. Basal ganglia/thalamus
      4. Brainstem
      5. Cerebellum
      6. Cranial nerves
      7. Spinal cord
      8. Spinal roots/peripheral nerves
      9. Ventricular system/CSF pathways
      10. Vascular system
      11. Neuromuscular junction/muscles
      12. Autonomic nervous system
      13. Embryology
      14. Pain pathways
      15. Radiologic anatomy/cerebral blood vessels (angiogram or magnetic resonance spectroscopy (MRA))
   B. Neuropathology
      1. Basic patterns of reaction
      2. Cerebrovascular disease
      3. Trauma (cranial and spinal)
      4. Metabolic/toxic/nutritional diseases
      5. Infections
      6. Demyelinating diseases/leukodystrophies
      7. Neoplasms
      8. Congenital/developmental disorders
      9. Degenerative/heterodegenerative disorders
      10. Myopathies
      11. Peripheral nerve disorders
      12. Radiologic pathology pertinent to assigned pathology sections
   C. Neurochemistry
      1. Carbohydrate metabolism
      2. Lipid metabolism
      3. Protein metabolism
      4. Neurotransmitters
      5. Axonal transport
      6. Energy metabolism

7. Blood–brain barrier
8. Biochemistry of membranes/ion channels
9. Neuronal excitation
10. Vitamins (general aspects)
11. Inborn errors of metabolism
12. Electrolytes and minerals
13. Neurotoxins
14. Free radical scavengers

D. Neurophysiology
  1. Basic
    a. Membrane physiology
    b. Synaptic transmission
    c. Sensory receptors and perception
    d. Special senses
    e. Reflexes
    f. Segmental and suprasegmental control of movement
    g. Cerebellar function
    h. Reticular system/mechanisms of sleep and arousal/consciousness/circadian rhythms
    i. Rhinencephalon/limbic system/visceral brain
    j. Learning and memory
    k. Cortical organizations and functions
    l. Pathophysiology of epilepsy
    m. Cerebral blood flow
    n. Autonomic function
    o. Blood–brain barrier
  2. Clinical
    a. Electroencephalogram (EEG)
    b. Evoked responses
    c. Electromyogram (EMG)/nerve conduction studies
    d. Sleep studies

E. Neuropharmacology
  1. Anticonvulsants
  2. Antibiotics/antimicrobials/vaccines
  3. Antioxidants
  4. Neuromuscular agents
  5. Antidyskinesia drugs (including antiparkinsonians)
  6. Vitamins (clinical aspects)
  7. Analgesics (non-narcotics, narcotics, and other centrally active agents)
  8. Anticoagulants/antiplatelets/thrombolytic agents
  9. Hormones
  10. Autonomic agents
  11. Anticholinesterase drugs
  12. Neurological side effects of systemic drugs
  13. Miscellaneous drugs

F. Neuroimmunology/Neurovirology
   1. Molecular pathogenesis of multiple sclerosis
   2. Molecular neurology of prion diseases and slow viruses
   3. Immunology in MS/MG/other neurological disorders
G. Neurogenetics/Molecular neurology and neuroepidemiology
   1. Mendelian-inherited diseases
   2. Mitochondrial disorders
   3. Trinucleotide repeat disorders
   4. Channelopathies
   5. Genetics of epilepsy
   6. Molecular genetics of brain tumors
   7. Other genetic disorders/mechanisms
   8. Ischemic penumbra
   9. Molecular approaches to stroke therapy
   10. Polymerase chain reaction
   11. Risk factors in neurological disease
   12. Demographics of neurological disease
H. Neuroendocrinology
I. Neuroimaging
   1. Plain skull/spine radiography
   2. MRI/MRV/MRS
   3. CT scan
   4. CT myelography
   5. Angiography
   6. SPECT/PET
J. Neuro-ophthalmology
   1. Vision and visual pathways
   2. Visual fields
   3. Pupils
   4. Ocular motility
   5. Fundi/retina/optic nerve
K. Neuro-otology
   1. Hearing/auditory function and testing
   2. Vertigo/vestibular function and testing
L. Cerebrospinal fluid
   1. Normal CSF constituents and volume
   2. Pathologic CSF patterns
      a. Cellular
      b. Chemical
      c. Enzymatic
      d. Serologic
M. Critical care and emergency medicine
N. Geriatric neurology
O. Headache and facial pain
P. Interventional neurology

Q. Movement disorders
R. Neurological rehabilitation

The discussion group judged all parts of this extensive list to be of the highest priority for neurologists, with the following caveats: neuro-ophthalmology was judged to be of slightly lower importance than the other topics, and neuroendocrinology, neuro-otology, and neurological rehabilitation were judged to be of lower importance than neuro-ophthalmology.

Sections of the outline were discussed essentially by outline letter grouping, but there was quite a bit of similarity in the outcomes of the discussions. All areas within the second neurology-specific Medical Knowledge Core Competency were considered for evaluation on the ABPN written certification (Part I) and/or oral certification (Part II) examinations with the exception of interventional neurology. The discussion group felt that topic should be covered only on the recertification examination, and even then, only the basic principles, not the techniques, should be covered. Regarding the rest of the outline, the discussion group did not specify which topics should be covered by which Part I and/or Part II examination. In addition, with the exception of neuroanatomy, neurophysiology, neuroimmunology/neurovirology, and geriatric neurology, all topics were designated for coverage on the recertification examination as well as the initial certification examination. Also, clinical neurophysiology, neuropharmacology, neuroimaging, neuro-ophthalmology, cerebral spinal fluid, critical care and emergency neurology, headache and facial pain, movement disorders, and neurological rehabilitation were listed as topics worthy of consideration on the Practice Assessment Component of the MOC Program.

Regarding the methodologies suggested for the assessment of this section of the outline, all areas, with the exception of critical care and emergency neurology, were suggested as suitable for MCQ testing. In addition, objective structured clinical examinations (OSCEs) were suggested as methodologies for evaluating neuropathology, clinical neurophysiology, neuroimaging, neuro-ophthalmology, neuro-otology, cerebral spinal fluid, and movement disorders; portfolios were suggested as means of evaluation for all of the same topics except movement disorders. Manual skills examinations were suggested for clinical neurophysiology, cerebral spinal fluid, and critical care and emergency neurology; virtual reality examinations were also suggested for critical care and emergency neurology.

DISCUSSION OF THE THIRD NEUROLOGY-SPECIFIC MEDICAL KNOWLEDGE CORE COMPETENCY

The third neurology-specific Medical Knowledge Core Competency is as follows:

3. *The physician shall demonstrate knowledge of patient evaluation and treatment selection, including:*
   A. The nature of patients' physical findings and the ability to correlate the findings with a likely localization for neurological dysfunction.

    B. Likely diagnoses and differential diagnoses
        1. In adults
        2. In children
    C. Planning for evaluation and management
    D. Potential risks and benefits of potential therapies, including surgical procedures
    E. Treatment comparison and selection

All of these topics were judged to be of the highest priority for evaluation. The discussion group believed these topics should be covered on the ABPN written certification (Part I) examination, the ABPN oral certification (Part II) examination, on the recertification examinations, and through the Practice Assessment Component of the ABPN MOC Program.

For this entire listing, the discussion group listed multiple choice examinations, in-training examinations, OSCEs, virtual reality examinations, and portfolios as suggested methodologies of assessment.

The discussion group believed that all neurology-specific Medical Knowledge Core Competencies could be validated by surveys of the field.

SUMMARY

The Medical Knowledge Core Competencies under discussion in this chapter (in abbreviated form) are as follows.

General Medical Knowledge Core Competencies

1. The physician shall demonstrate knowledge of the major disorders, including the following:
   A. The epidemiology of the disorder.
   B. The etiology of the disorder, including medical, genetic, and social factors.
   C. The phenomenology of the disorder.
   D. Diagnostic criteria.
   E. Effective treatment strategies.
   F. Course and prognosis.
2. The physician shall demonstrate knowledge of healthcare delivery systems
3. The physician shall demonstrate knowledge of ethics in neurology/psychiatry.
4. The physician shall demonstrate the ability to reference and utilize electronic information systems to access medical, scientific, and patient information.

Neurology-Specific Medical Knowledge Core Competencies

1. The physician shall demonstrate knowledge of basic neuroscience that would be critical to the practice of neurology, including cognitive, behavioral, and social development.

2. The physician shall demonstrate knowledge of major neurological and psychiatric disorders and familiarity with the scientific basis of neurological diseases, including the following:
   A. Neuroanatomy.
   B. Neuropathology.
   C. Neurochemistry.
   D. Neurophysiology.
   E. Neuropharmacology.
   F. Neuroimmunology/Neurovirology.
   G. Neurogenetics/Molecular neurology and neuroepidemiology.
   H. Neuroendocrinology.
   I. Neuroimaging.
   J. Neuro-ophthalmology.
   K. Neuro-otology.
   L. Cerebrospinal fluid.
   M. Critical care and emergency medicine.
   N. Geriatric neurology.
   O. Headache and facial pain.
   P. Interventional neurology.
   Q. Movement disorders.
   R. Neurological rehabilitation.
3. The physician shall demonstrate knowledge of patient evaluation and treatment selection, including:
   A. The nature of patients' physical findings and the ability to correlate the findings with a likely localization for neurological dysfunction.
   B. Likely diagnoses and differential diagnoses:
      1. In adults
      2. In children
   C. Planning for evaluation and management.
   D. Potential risks and benefits of potential therapies, including surgical procedures.
   E. Treatment comparison and selection.

To summarize, the Medical Knowledge section of the core competency outline as discussed at the ABPN Invitational Core Competencies Conference is divided into three sections: a general section, a neurology-specific section, and a psychiatry-specific section. Only the first two sections are discussed here. Psychiatry core competencies will be covered in Chapter 11 of this book, which will deal with what neurologists need to know about psychiatry for their clinical practice.

All of the core competencies in the Medical Knowledge section of the outline were judged to be of highest priority in terms of assessment, with the exception of the following:

- Knowledge of healthcare delivery systems (the second core competency in the general section), which was judged to be of low priority for assessment purposes.

- The ability to reference and use electronic information systems to access medical, scientific, and patient information (the fourth core competency in the general section), which the group did not believe warranted assessment at this time.
- Knowledge of neuro-ophthalmology, neuroendocrinology, neuro-otology, and neurological rehabilitation (portions of the second neurology-specific core competency).

For all Medical Knowledge Core Competencies, it was felt that the residency program faculty would be key teachers in assisting their residents to master these core competencies. As with any educational setting, feedback during the learning process here would be important so that remediation, when needed, could occur. Formal assessment of these competencies would be done by the ABPN for initial certification and on the recertification examinations. In addition, most of these competencies could also be evaluated under the Practice Assessment Component of the ABPN MOC Program. Portfolio assessment of most of these competencies would also be a possibility.

All of the Medical Knowledge Core Competencies could be validated by surveys of the field to determine that they are, in fact, core competencies for neurologists.

NOTES

1. Discussion of this neurology-specific core competency after the conference condensed this competency to what is listed here as the capital letters of the outline.

7

Interpersonal and Communications Skills Core Competencies

José Biller, M.D.

ASSUMPTIONS REGARDING THE SIX CATEGORIES OF CORE COMPETENCIES

The core competencies under discussion in this book are divided into six categories:

- Patient Care
- Medical Knowledge
- Interpersonal and Communications Skills
- Practice-Based Learning and Improvement
- Professionalism
- Systems-Based Practice

The first two categories of core competencies, Patient Care (discussed in Chapter 5) and Medical Knowledge (discussed in Chapter 6) are alike in that they are each divided into three sections: a general section, a neurology-specific section, and a psychiatry-specific section. In each of the preceding two chapters, only the general and neurology-specific sections were discussed. To the extent necessary, the core competencies that are psychiatry-specific will be discussed in the chapter on cross-competencies (Chapter 11). The focus therein will be on what neurologists need to know about psychiatry.

At the American Board of Psychiatry and Neurology (ABPN) Invitational Conference on Core Competencies, there was consensus that the first two categories of core competencies (Patient Care and Medical Knowledge) would need to have specialty-specific components in addition to a general category. Unlike those two categories of core competencies, consensus was also that it was likely that the next four categories of core competencies (Interpersonal and Communication Skills, Practice-Based Learning and Improvement, Professionalism, and Systems-Based Practice) would probably contain competencies that would be (or could be) applicable to most medical specialties.

If it were to be the case that the last four categories of core competencies would be either the same or similar for most medical specialties, the American Board of Medical Specialties (ABMS) could assist the twenty-four specialty Boards in coordinating efforts to define the specific competencies for these areas. With this possible future endeavor, it is anticipated that the ABMS will work closely with its member Boards that have already attempted delineation of these categories.

With this rationale, this chapter on Interpersonal and Communications Skills and the three following it (Chapter 8, Practice-Based Learning and Improvement; Chapter 9, Professionalism; and Chapter 10, Systems-Based Practice) will assume less of a neurology-specific view and more of a global view of medical core competencies.

ASSUMPTIONS REGARDING THE INTERPERSONAL AND COMMUNICATIONS SKILLS CORE COMPETENCIES

As the physician/patient relationship is central to any healthcare program, it is logical that the core competencies in the Interpersonal and Communication Skills Category are of great importance. Therefore, it was assumed that the majority of competencies listed in this category would be of highest priority for assessment purposes. Those rated differently will be discussed as they arise in the listing below.

It was generally assumed that almost all of these competencies should be assessed through oral examinations using either actual or standardized patients; it was also assumed that the majority of these competencies should be evaluated under the Practice Assessment Component of the ABPN Maintenance of Certification (MOC) Program.

ABOUT THE DISCUSSION BELOW

During the discussion of this section of the core competency outline, essentially every point and subpoint were discussed separately. For the sake of presentation here, points which follow one another will be discussed together when the discussion of them is either the same or similar. Important differences will be noted.

DISCUSSION OF POINTS A THROUGH C OF THE FIRST INTERPERSONAL AND COMMUNICATIONS SKILLS CORE COMPETENCY

The grouping of core competencies that can be said to comprise the first Interpersonal and Communications Skills Core Competency is as follows:

1. *The physician shall demonstrate the following abilities:*
   A. To listen to and understand patients.

B. To communicate effectively with patients using verbal, non-verbal, and written skills as appropriate.
C. To develop and maintain a therapeutic alliance with patients by instilling feelings of trust, openness, rapport, and comfort in the relationship with the physician.

This grouping of core competencies could be evaluated on oral examinations using points similar to the ABPN oral certification (Part II) examination. The discussion group decided that this was already being done adequately for Points A and B above, but inadequately for Point C. It was also thought that all three points should be evaluated under the Practice Assessment Component of the ABPN MOC Program.

Generally, in oral examinations with actual or standardized patients, the patients are not asked to rate the physicians (residents or ABPN certification candidates). Gathering information from the patients, however, could be a viable option for the future as long as what the patients were asked to rate was under the patients' purview. Thus, it would be logical that patients could rate residents or ABPN certification candidates on Points A and B above. Patients could express their opinions as to whether or not the physician seemed to listen to and understand them and if the physician communicated effectively (from the patient's point of view). In fact, no one other than the patients can rate what they thought about these two issues. External raters, such as program directors or examiners, could also rate the physician/patient encounters, but the best judge of these two points would probably be the patients themselves.

This situation is, however, not true for Point C. Patients could not be logically asked to ascertain if therapeutic alliances had been developed and maintained. Patients could report on the establishment of rapport, but not on the creation of therapeutic alliances. This evaluation would have to be done by a medically qualified external person, most likely a physician observer.

The discussion group thought that an external reviewer could validate these three related competencies.

DISCUSSION OF POINTS D THROUGH F OF THE FIRST INTERPERSONAL AND COMMUNICATIONS SKILLS CORE COMPETENCY

The next grouping of items under the first Interpersonal and Communications Skills Core Competency is as follows:

1. (continued) *The physician shall demonstrate the following abilities:*
   D. To use negotiation to develop an agreed upon healthcare management plan with patients.
   E. To transmit information to patients in a clear, meaningful fashion.
   F. To understand the impact of the physician's own feelings and behavior on treatment.

Point D above was judged to be of less importance than the preceding three Points (A, B, and C) or Points E and F listed above. Also, the discussion group decided that Point D, the physician's skill in negotiating a healthcare management plan with patients, could be assessed using multiple choice questions (MCQs), especially those of the branching variety. Such MCQs would have to be very carefully worded. Oral examinations could also be used to assess negotiation skills.

The discussion group decided that Points E and F, the physician's abilities to transmit information to patients and to understand the impact of one's own feelings and behavior on the treatment, could be best assessed using some type of oral interview or patient observation process, most likely using vignettes or objective structured clinical examinations (OSCEs). It was decided that all three points above could and should be evaluated under the Practice Assessment Component of the ABPN MOC Program. This evaluation would also serve as the validation for these skills.

Consistent with the discussion above, the group decided that the negotiating skills of a physician (Point D) could be assessed using branching logic questions, for example, on an MCQ examination. Points E and F above would be better assessed using vignettes or OSCEs. Testing the extent to which a physician understands the impact of one's own feelings and behavior on treatment for the patient could also be assessed in an oral examination.

DISCUSSION OF POINTS G THROUGH I OF THE FIRST INTERPERSONAL AND COMMUNICATIONS SKILLS CORE COMPETENCY

The next grouping of items under the first Interpersonal and Communications Skills Core Competency is as follows:

1. (continued) *The physician shall demonstrate the following abilities:*
   G. To communicate effectively and work collaboratively with allied healthcare professionals and with other professionals involved in the lives of patients.
   H. To educate patients, professionals, and the public about medical, psychological, and behavioral issues.
   I. To work effectively within multidisciplinary team structures as member, consultant, or leader.

Of these three points, the first listed above – the physician's ability to work collaboratively with a healthcare team of professionals – was thought to be of higher priority than the other two skills.

In discussion, the group saw similarities between Point G and I in that they would both require some type of oral assessment for initial certification purposes and would also require evaluation under the Practice Assessment Component of the ABPN MOC Program. The group also thought both vignettes and OSCEs would be suitable methodologies for assessing competence for these skills.

Point H, the physician's ability to educate patients, professionals, and the public about medical, psychological, and social issues, was clearly seen as a skill that develops slowly over the individual professional's life from residency into and through practice. A physician in residency training or even in early practice could not be expected to have this skill to any measurable level. This is clearly a skill that develops with experience and maturity. The discussion group believed that the physician should be held accountable under the Lifelong Learning Component of the ABPN MOC Program to show evidence of study to have the current information to be able to communicate to patients and others. The process of communicating that information or of educating others could be assessed through oral examinations, vignettes, and OSCEs. The group decided that this particular skill should be documented under both the Lifelong Learning Component and the Practice Assessment Component of the ABPN MOC Program.

DISCUSSION OF THE SECOND INTERPERSONAL AND COMMUNICATIONS SKILLS CORE COMPETENCY

The second Interpersonal and Communications Skills Core Competency is as follows:

2. *The physician shall demonstrate the ability to elicit important diagnostic data and data affecting treatment from individuals from the full spectrum of ethnic, racial, gender, and educational backgrounds. This will include skills in tolerating and managing highly charged affect in patients.*

This competency, rated at the highest priority, clearly has training implications that can be assessed almost continuously throughout residency. Assessment of this multi-faceted competency could be done through MCQs, oral interviews using either actual or standardized patients, vignettes, and OSCEs. The discussion group clearly saw this competency as needing evaluation under the Practice Assessment Component of the ABPN MOC Program.

DISCUSSION OF THE THIRD INTERPERSONAL AND COMMUNICATIONS SKILLS CORE COMPETENCY

The third Interpersonal and Communications Skills Core Competency is as follows:

3. *The physician shall demonstrate the ability to obtain, interpret, and evaluate consultations from other medical specialties. This shall include:*
   A. Knowing when to solicit consultation and having sensitivity to assess the need for consultation.
   B. Discussing the consultation findings with patients and their families.
   C. Evaluating the consultation findings.

The three skills listed as parts of this competency are clearly related, and the group saw them as being of the highest importance. All skills could be assessed through simple MCQs and oral interviews. Other methodologies suggested for use in evaluating these skills included branching logic questions, vignettes, and OSCEs. All skills could be validated through the Practice Assessment Component of the ABPN MOC Program.

DISCUSSION OF THE FOURTH INTERPERSONAL AND COMMUNICATIONS SKILLS CORE COMPETENCY

The fourth Interpersonal and Communications Skills Core Competency is as follows:

4. *The physician shall serve as an effective consultant to other medical specialists, mental health professionals, and community agencies. The physician shall demonstrate the ability to:*
   A. Communicate effectively with the requesting party to refine the consultation question.
   B. Maintain the role of consultant.
   C. Communicate clear and specific recommendations.
   D. Respect the knowledge and expertise of the requesting party.

The related skills of this competency were judged to be of the highest priority for assessment purposes. They could be assessed using MCQs, oral interviews, vignettes, OSCEs, and branching logic questions. The discussion group saw these skills as needing evaluation under the Practice Assessment Component of the ABPN MOC Program.

DISCUSSION OF THE FIFTH INTERPERSONAL AND COMMUNICATIONS SKILLS CORE COMPETENCY

The fifth Interpersonal and Communications Skills Core Competency is as follows:

5. *The physician shall demonstrate the ability to communicate effectively with patients and their families by:*
   A. Gearing all communication to the educational/intellectual levels of patients and their families.
   B. Demonstrating cultural sensitivity to patients and their families.
   C. Providing explanations of neurological and psychiatric disorders and treatment (both verbally and in written form) that are jargon-free and geared to the educational/intellectual level of patients and their families.
   D. Providing preventive education that is understandable and practical.
   E. Respecting the patients' cultural, ethnic, and economic backgrounds.

F. Developing and enhancing rapport and a working alliance with patients and their families.

G. Assuring that patients and their families understand what is being communicated.

These related skills were thought, similar to most others in this category, to be of the highest priority for assessment purposes. The discussion group saw these skills as being assessed through MCQs, oral examinations, OSCEs, and branching logic questions. They also saw these skills as being able to be validated through the Practice Assessment Component of the ABPN MOC Program.

DISCUSSION OF THE SIXTH INTERPERSONAL AND COMMUNICATIONS SKILLS CORE COMPETENCY

The sixth Interpersonal and Communications Skills Core Competency is as follows:

6. *The physician shall maintain medical records and written prescriptions that are legible and up to date. These records must capture essential information while simultaneously respecting patient privacy and be useful to health professionals outside neurology and psychiatry.*

This core competency is unlike most of the other competencies discussed in this and other sections of the outline in that it is clearly a practice issue. While residents can be taught to create records that are legible, it takes an on-going practice to assess how current the records are, how well the records respect the patient's privacy, and if the records are useful to other medical professionals. Thus, this competency, judged to be of priority importance, can only be evaluated as part of the Practice Assessment Component of the ABPN MOC Program.

DISCUSSION OF THE SEVENTH INTERPERSONAL AND COMMUNICATIONS SKILLS CORE COMPETENCY

The seventh Interpersonal and Communications Skills Core Competency is as follows:

7. *The physician shall demonstrate the ability to effectively lead a multidisciplinary treatment team, including being able to:*
    A. Listen effectively.
    B. Elicit needed information from team members.
    C. Integrate information from different disciplines.
    D. Manage conflict.
    E. Clearly communicate an integrated treatment plan.
    F. Maintain a singularity of purpose for the coordination of patient care.
    G. Coordinate efforts to eliminate or minimize medical errors.

This competency represents a skill set of secondary importance; effectively leading a multidisciplinary team is clearly secondary to practicing excellent medicine. It is, nonetheless, an important skill, one which residents can learn and practice during training and one which mature, well-established physicians in some specialties practice daily. Like the core competency immediately preceding it, this skill can really only be evaluated as part of the Practice Assessment Component of the ABPN MOC Program.

DISCUSSION OF THE EIGHTH INTERPERSONAL AND COMMUNICATIONS SKILLS CORE COMPETENCY

The eighth Interpersonal and Communications Skills Core Competency is as follows:

8. *The physician shall demonstrate the ability to communicate effectively with patients and their families while respecting confidentiality. Such communication may include:*
   A. The results of the assessment.
   B. Use of informed consent when ordering investigative procedures.
   C. Genetic counseling and palliative care when appropriate.
   D. Consideration and compassion for the patient in providing accurate medical information and prognosis.
   E. The risks and benefits of the proposed treatment plan, including possible side-effects of medications and/or treatments.
   F. Alternatives (if any) to the proposed treatment plan.
   G. Education concerning the disorder, its prognosis, and prevention strategies.

This important communication skill was judged to be of the highest priority. The discussion group saw this competency as needing to be evaluated at multiple points in a physician's training and career. They decided that this skill set could be assessed through well-written MCQs, oral examinations, vignettes, and OSCEs. The discussion group also saw this skill set as being assessed under three components of the ABPN MOC Program: in the Lifelong Learning Component, on the Recertification Examination, and through Practice Assessment.

Validation of the skills comprising this core competency could be validated through the Practice Assessment Component of the ABPN MOC Program, through outcome studies (for points A through D listed above), and by self-reporting (for point E through G above).

SUMMARY

The full outline of Interpersonal and Communication Skills Core Competencies is listed below:

1. The physician shall demonstrate the following abilities:
   A. To listen to and understand patients.

  B. To communicate effectively with patients, using verbal, non-verbal, and written skills as appropriate.

  C. To develop and maintain a therapeutic alliance with patients by instilling feelings of trust, openness, rapport, and comfort in the relationship with the physician.

  D. To use negotiation to develop an agreed upon healthcare management plan with patients.

  E. To transmit information to patients in a clear, meaningful fashion.

  F. To understand the impact of the physician's own feelings and behavior on treatment.

  G. To communicate effectively and work collaboratively with allied healthcare professionals and with other professionals involved in the lives of patients.

  H. To educate patients, professionals, and the public about medical, psychological, and behavioral issues.

  I. To work effectively within multidisciplinary team structures as member, consultant, or leader.

2. The physician shall demonstrate the ability to elicit important diagnostic data and data affecting treatment from individuals from the full spectrum of ethnic, racial, gender, and educational backgrounds. This will include skills in tolerating and managing highly charged affect in patients.

3. The physician shall demonstrate the ability to obtain, interpret, and evaluate consultations from other medical specialties. This shall include:

  A. Knowing when to solicit consultation and having sensitivity to assess the need for consultation.

  B. Discussing the consultation findings with patients and their families.

  C. Evaluating the consultation findings.

4. The physician shall serve as an effective consultant to other medical specialists, mental health professionals, and community agencies. The physician shall demonstrate the abilities to:

  A. Communicate effectively with the requesting party to refine the consultation question.

  B. Maintain the role of consultant.

  C. Communicate clear and specific recommendations.

  D. Respect the knowledge and expertise of the requesting party.

5. The physician shall demonstrate the ability to communicate effectively with patients and their families by:

  A. Gearing all communication to the educational/intellectual levels of patients and their families.

  B. Demonstrating cultural sensitivity to patients and their families.

  C. Providing explanations of neurological and psychiatric disorders and treatment (both verbally and in written form) that are jargon-free and geared to the educational/intellectual level of patients and their families.

    D. Providing preventive education that is understandable and practical.

    E. Respecting the patients' cultural, ethnic, and economic backgrounds.

    F. Developing and enhancing rapport and a working alliance with patients and their families.

    G. Assuring that patients and their families understand what is being communicated.

6. The physician shall maintain medical records and written prescriptions that are legible and up to date. These records must capture essential information while simultaneously respecting patient privacy and be useful to health professionals outside neurology and psychiatry.

7. The physician shall demonstrate the ability to effectively lead a multidisciplinary treatment team, including being able to:

    A. Listen effectively.

    B. Elicit needed information from team members.

    C. Integrate information from different disciplines.

    D. Manage conflict.

    E. Clearly communicate an integrated treatment plan.

    F. Maintain a singularity of purpose for the coordination of patient care.

    G. Coordinate efforts to eliminate or minimize medical errors.

8. The physician shall demonstrate the ability to communicate effectively with patients and their families while respecting confidentiality. Such communication may include:

    A. The results of the assessment.

    B. Use of informed consent when ordering investigative procedures.

    C. Genetic counseling and palliative care when appropriate.

    D. Consideration and compassion for the patient in providing accurate medical information and prognosis.

    E. The risks and benefits of the proposed treatment plan, including possible side-effects of medications and/or treatments.

    F. Alternatives (if any) to the proposed treatment plan.

    G. Education concerning the disorder, its prognosis, and prevention strategies.

The Interpersonal and Communications Skills Core Competency Category of the outline represents the first to be described that could be said to be essentially common across all specialties. While the items above came from the work of specific specialty groups, it is anticipated that other specialty groups would come up with essentially the same list of competencies.

All of the skills comprising the competencies in this section were judged to be of highest importance, except for those skills that involved negotiating healthcare maintenance plans, educating patients and others, and working as part of or leading a team of other health professionals. It is not that these skills are unimportant; these skills are of secondary importance and can be assessed after the more essential skills have been addressed. A more valid assessment of these skills may also be possible only after the physician has had some time to develop them in practice.

While the discussion group suggested MCQs as evaluation tools for many of the skills within this section of competencies, it must be remembered that MCQs assessing interpersonal and communications skills are difficult to write. Far more logical for the evaluation of these skills would be oral examinations, observations of physician/patient interactions, vignettes, and OSCEs. For a limited number of these skills, assessment could be handled by consulting with the person receiving the communication whether that would be a patient, a nurse, another physician, or another health professional. Interpersonal and communications skills can effectively be evaluated at the same time other core competencies are evaluated.

The core competencies listed in this area are worthy of constant assessment from residency training and all through practice.

8

Practice-Based Learning and Improvement Core Competencies

Michael V. Johnston, M.D.

DISCUSSION OF PRACTICE-BASED LEARNING AND IMPROVEMENT CORE COMPETENCIES VIS-À-VIS THE OTHER CORE COMPETENCY CATEGORIES

The Practice-Based Learning and Improvement Core Competency Category is different from the three previous Categories. The focus of this competency area is the practicing physician, and more specifically the learning and improvement that comes to the physician through practice. The goal of this section is to stress planned, purposeful learning without discounting natural or serendipitous learning. This section of core competencies attempts to capitalize on all learning and structure it into a formal pattern that will benefit the individual physician and the patient population being served.

This section of core competencies relates directly to the Maintenance of Certification (MOC) Program©, which the American Board of Medical Specialties (ABMS) is proposing to take the place of just a recertification examination. At one time not very many years ago, Board certification was seen as the ultimate achievement for a physician. There was no formal plan for continuing the physician's education after certification; it was assumed that a physician would learn what was needed when it was needed and would do so by choice.

Medicine has always been a dynamic field, but never more so than right now. Medical knowledge is expanding at such a phenomenal rate that it is not humanly possible to keep up with all of the latest developments. Yet it is imperative that physicians stay up to date with new knowledge. The ABMS, working through its specialty Boards, has taken steps to guarantee medical learning after physician practice has begun.

Specialty Boards, at the urging of the ABMS, are all moving to "time-limited certification," which means that a physician, once initially Board-certified, will remain certified only for a specified number of years. For neurologists, this period is ten years. After the initial ten-year period of certification, the neurologist will have to become certified again ("recertified") by taking a cognitive examination similar to the initial certification examination. This new development was not necessarily well received by younger physicians who claimed that they were being discriminated against compared to what had been allowed for more senior physicians. For better or for worse, the senior physicians' certification could not be changed after their having earned "lifetime certification;" rules can not be changed after the fact.

The cry of "unfair treatment" became louder when the ABMS mandated that not only was a recertification examination to be required, but that the examination would have to be a secure, proctored examination as opposed to a take-home recertification examination to be completed at leisure. This mandate for a secure, proctored examination was made at the request of the state licensing boards and institutions which demanded assurance that the person taking the examination was, in fact, that person and not an imposter.

After reflection, the ABMS decided that a cognitive examination, occupying perhaps four hours each decade, did not seem to be enough to guarantee that physicians were up to date. They opined that the recertification examination needed to be a part of a larger program; thus, the Maintenance of Certification (MOC) Program© was designed.

As envisioned by the ABMS, the MOC Program© would have four components, with the second listed here being directly related to the Practice-Based Learning and Improvement Core Competency Category being discussed in this chapter. The four components of the ABMS MOC Program© are as follows:

1. Evidence of Professional Standing.
2. Evidence of Lifelong Learning and Periodic Self-Assessment.
3. Evidence of Cognitive Expertise.
4. Evidence of Evaluations of Practice Performance.

The first requirement of the MOC Program© – Evidence of Professional Standing – is neither new nor surprising. The American Board of Psychiatry and Neurology (ABPN) has always had this requirement of evidence of professional standing. Evidence has taken the form of the requirement of a full, unrestricted medical license, with documentation to be provided at the time of registration for a certification examination. This requirement has been in effect since 1935 for initial certification examinations, and since 2000 when the first recertification examinations were offered. There is currently no plan for the ABPN to change this requirement.

The second requirement of the MOC Program© – Evidence of Lifelong Learning and Periodic Self-Assessment – relates directly to the Practice-Based Learning and Improvement Core Competency Category of the outline. While the rest of the chapter will explore this relationship, it is of value now to look at the component parts of this section of the MOC Program©. The ABMS guidelines specify that evidence of lifelong learning and periodic self-assessment will require the following:

- Documentation of participation in specialty-specific educational activities.
- Documentation of participation in specialty-specific self-assessment activities.

- A relationship between the lifelong learning activities and performance standards.

This section contains some interesting aspects. Among them are the following:

- This section of the MOC Program© speaks of "lifelong learning." Thus, it is assumed that physicians, simply by their status as physicians, will be committed to some form of learning throughout life.
- This section of the MOC Program© speaks of documentation of participation in educational activities. This implies that the learning a physician will undertake while in practice cannot be serendipitous, haphazard, or left to chance. The learning must constitute some form of organized activity, which of its nature implies both structure and goals. The discussion group indicated that it would be most beneficial if such educational activities were structured into some type of program.
- The use of the word "participation" is interesting, in that for most Continuing Medical Education (CME) Programs, "participation" is generally judged by simply being present in the room where the activity is taking place. (Sometimes not even that is required. The signing in at the beginning of the activity or the payment of a registration fee suffices for enough "participation" to earn a CME certificate in some cases.) It is possible that the ABPN and its sister Boards may choose to define "participation" in terms of some form of assessment that demonstrates that learning has actually occurred. Pre- and post-tests can measure cognitive gain, but generally the documentation of participation in the educational activity is in no way tied to the achievement on the post-test.
- The MOC Program© notes that the educational activities must be "specialty-specific." This indicates that participation in a serendipitous array of activities will not suffice. Most of the lifelong learning required here would probably emanate from relevant specialty societies. Some ABMS Boards already require that a stated number of specialty-specific CME hours be documented prior to a diplomate taking a recertification examination.
- Besides being "specialty-specific," the discussion group also thought that the educational activities should be "relevant." "Specialty-specific" is certainly clear, but "relevant" is more ambiguous, as one must determine relevance in relationship to what? Certainly, the continuing medical education should be relevant to the specialty, but relevance also relates to the physician participating in the activity. Most likely, relevance would be determined by use of self-assessment examinations as discussed below.
- Linking self-assessment programs to member Board certification requirements appears to provide the clarity needed for determining and designing a *specialty-specific* and *relevant* continuing medical education *program*. This means, of course, that member Boards must have a self-assessment program linked to their certification requirements. As most ABMS member Boards are not, and do not want to be, involved in education – even at the self-assessment level – this requirement also

seems to offer an opportunity for the member Boards to partner with their appropriate specialty societies to meet this requirement.

The third requirement of the MOC Program© – the recertification examination – has been discussed earlier. This cognitive examination, in a multiple-choice question (MCQ) format, is meant to ascertain (to the degree such an examination can do so) that the physician is practicing medicine consistent with current medical knowledge and up-to-date treatment practices. While the recertification examination could certainly retest basic science and other topics covered on the initial certification examination, the ABPN plans for its specialty and subspecialty recertification examinations to focus on practice issues. This is consistent with the specifications of the ABMS that the recertification examination focus on current knowledge of clinical science and that it be relevant to maintenance of certification.

The fourth requirement of the MOC Program© – assessment of practice-based performance – is the specialty board's commitment to assuring that the physicians' patterns of practice meet acceptable standards. The specialty Boards, with the support of the ABMS, are currently undertaking measures to determine how and when this assessment should take place and what its exact nature or form will be. This part of the ABPN MOC Program will probably not be available for implementation until later in this decade.

ASSUMPTIONS REGARDING THE PRACTICE-BASED LEARNING AND IMPROVEMENT CORE COMPETENCIES

As explained by its title and in the discussion above, it is logical to assume that core competencies in the Practice-Based Learning and Improvement Category of the core competency outline will be assessed at specified points during a physician's practice as part of the mandated MOC Program©. Thus, it can also be assumed that most, if not all, of the core competencies of this section will not have relevance for assessment purposes during residency or at the time of initial certification. Residency training, done well, would lay an excellent groundwork for these competencies to be established and maintained during practice.

A second assumption is that because the focus of the Practice-Based Learning and Improvement Core Competencies is on the period of practice (as opposed to the period of residency), the assessment of these core competencies would most aptly be part of the Lifelong Learning and Practice-Based Assessment Components of the MOC Program©.

DISCUSSION OF THE FIRST PRACTICE-BASED LEARNING AND IMPROVEMENT CORE COMPETENCY

During the ABPN Invitational Core Competencies Conference, each subpoint of the sections of the Practice-Based Learning and Improvement outline was discussed separately. That is how the points will be presented here with groupings occurring only when discussion of them was essentially similar. Subpoints of the competencies listed for discussion below do not imply that they are of lesser importance than other main points.

The first Practice-Based Learning and Improvement Core Competency is as follows:

1. *The physician shall recognize limitations in his or her own knowledge base and clinical skills, and understand and address the need for lifelong learning.*

The discussion group concurred that in addition to recognizing and accepting the limitations of personal knowledge, a physician must also acknowledge the need for continued learning and the importance of conferring with other specialists and healthcare providers when the situation warrants. This is critical for optimum patient care. For this reason especially, this competency was seen to be of highest priority.

The discussion group believed that this competency could initially be assessed during oral interviews, such as are held in residency and as part of the ABPN oral certification (Part II) examination. Special vignettes could be written for this purpose.

This competency should also receive additional assessment during the Lifelong Learning and Practice Assessment Components of the ABPN MOC Program. Exactly how this competency would be assessed at those times was not discussed at length, but it would be logical to assume that a physician's lack of knowledge in a given area would be the motivating force behind a continuing medical education program. A database of continuing medical education activities and of patient practice would be helpful for this assessment.

It is also logical to assume that an analysis of practice patterns would indicate where a physician decided that his knowledge, skills, or specialty would be insufficient to treat a given patient; that would then be the point where other specialists or healthcare providers would be called in. Assessment of this practice component might be handled with 360-degree evaluations (evaluations done by multiple people in a person's sphere of influence, usually superiors, peers, subordinates, and patients and their families).

DISCUSSION OF THE SECOND PRACTICE-BASED LEARNING AND IMPROVEMENT CORE COMPETENCY

The second Practice-Based Learning and Improvement Core Competency is as follows:

2. *The physician shall demonstrate appropriate skills for obtaining up-to-date information from scientific and practice literature and other sources to assist in the quality care of patients. This shall include, but not be limited to, the following:*
A. Use of medical libraries.

B. Use of information technology, including Internet-based searches and literature databases (e.g., Medline).
C. Use of drug information databases.

This competency would be of critical importance to the Lifelong Learning Component of the ABPN MOC Program. Of the three points above, the discussion group agreed that the ability to use information technology like the Internet was more critical than the other two points. It is, of course, logical to assume that specialists – especially those in large practices – would not have to perform literature searches on their own, but they should always have the knowledge of how such searches are done in order to direct the work of those doing the Internet work. The discussion group decided that using case-based vignettes that would require library or other research would be an excellent methodology for assessing this competency.

DISCUSSION OF THE THIRD PRACTICE-BASED LEARNING AND IMPROVEMENT CORE COMPETENCY

The third Practice-Based Learning and Improvement Core Competency is as follows:

3. *The physician shall demonstrate appropriate skills for obtaining up-to-date information from scientific and practice literature and other sources to assist in the quality care of patients. This shall include, but not be limited to, the active participation, as appropriate, in educational courses, conferences, and other organized educational activities both at the local and national levels.*

This competency directly ties into the Lifelong Learning Component of the MOC Program. It is, in fact, the basis for the current CME infrastructure, that is, of a physician attending and *participating actively* in educational programs. In discussion, there were a number of criticisms of the current CME situation. These included the following:

- Physicians self-select their own CME activities. It is assumed that the selection is based on need, but currently there is no way to link attendance and participation at CME events to any type of individual physician needs assessment. In order for the learning from these educational programs to be meaningful for the purposes of this competency, the learning must answer a specific need. This need could be real or perceived, but would require being measured and documented. Various needs assessment processes could be used; these might include, but not be limited to, specialty-specific self-assessments, normed assessments, and mentor-assisted assessments.

- Left to one's own devices, most people will choose to learn more about favorite subjects or participate in activities in which they already have some degree of proficiency. Thus, areas in which a deficit of knowledge, a lack of skills, or a troublesome attitude is present may be those areas specifically NOT selected for CME or other educational activities. In that case, the learning that comes about because of the selection of a particular educational activity is really an enhancement of an already adequate area, not the meeting of a true need.
- CME activities are currently measured in credit hours. A physician earns one CME credit hour for each hour spent attending an educational program. Thus, the currency is "seat-time," and not a measure of learning. While seat-time might still be the currency used for measurement, this core competency demands that the change in knowledge, skills, or attitudes based on the educational activity be measured and documented.
- The discussion group especially recommended that CME be specialty-specific to ensure that meaningful learning is taking place.

DISCUSSION OF THE FOURTH PRACTICE-BASED LEARNING AND IMPROVEMENT CORE COMPETENCY

The fourth Practice-Based Learning and Improvement Core Competency is as follows:

4. *The physician shall evaluate caseload and practice experience in a systematic manner. This may include case-based learning.*

This core competency, and also the ones immediately following, ask physicians to evaluate themselves according to various parameters. The wording of this competency prompted some discussion. Questions asked included the following:

- Will the evaluation be accomplished by physicians doing a self-assessment by an outside agent or group?
- What should be done with the results of that assessment?
- If there is no follow-up from the assessment, what is the point of doing it?
- How can or should such an evaluation (and follow-up measures) be documented?
- What does "systematic" mean in this core competency? Who establishes the system? The physician? The specialty? Another agency?
- If this core competency is to be considered as part of the MOC Program, would not that imply that someone other than physicians themselves should be doing the assessment? And, if another does the assessment of the physician, the questions in other bullets still remain to be answered.

While these questions were not specifically answered, the fact that they were raised at all speaks to how difficult assessing the core competencies in this section of the outline will be. It also points out the same difficulties for standards to be set to address the Lifelong Learning Component of a MOC Program.

The discussion group did suggest that evidence would be needed that the physician has participated in some type of certified case-based quality assurance program. They suggested further that it might be the specialty societies, such as the American Academy of Neurology (AAN), who should undertake this task.

DISCUSSION OF THE FIFTH PRACTICE-BASED LEARNING AND IMPROVEMENT CORE COMPETENCY

The fifth Practice-Based Learning and Improvement Core Competency is as follows:

5. *The physician shall evaluate caseload and practice experience in a systematic manner. This may include, but not be limited to the following:*
   A. Use of best practices through practice guidelines or clinical pathways.
   B. Review of patient records and outcomes.
   C. Obtaining evaluations from patients (e.g., outcomes and patient satisfaction).

The discussion group saw clearly that this competency, including its subpoints, should be part of the Lifelong Learning and Practice Assessment Components of the ABPN MOC Program. The use of best practices through practice guidelines or clinical pathways could also be evaluated during oral interviews, such as the ABPN oral certification (Part II) examination, using specially designed case vignettes. The discussion group suggested that specialty societies might find meaningful ways to assist with the assessment of the review of patient records and outcomes and obtaining evaluations from patients.

DISCUSSION OF THE SIXTH PRACTICE-BASED LEARNING AND IMPROVEMENT CORE COMPETENCY

The sixth Practice-Based Learning and Improvement Core Competency is as follows:

6. *The physician shall evaluate caseload and practice experience in a systematic manner. This may include, but not be limited to, the following:*
   A. Obtaining appropriate supervision and consultation.

B. Maintaining a system for examining errors in practice and initiating improvements to eliminate or reduce errors.

Unlike most of the core competencies in the Practice-Based Learning and Improvement Category of the outline, both subpoints of this core competency were rated as being of highest priority. Both subpoints could be evaluated under the Lifelong Learning and Self-Assessment Component of a MOC Program, but could probably be evaluated more completely under the Practice Assessment Component of a MOC Program. The discussion group suggested a third-party evaluation for both subpoints with benchmarks being established by the ABPN.

DISCUSSION OF THE SEVENTH PRACTICE-BASED LEARNING AND IMPROVEMENT CORE COMPETENCY

The seventh Practice-Based Learning and Improvement Core Competency is as follows:

7. *The physician shall demonstrate an ability to critically evaluate relevant medical literature. This ability may include using knowledge of common methodologies employed in neurological and psychiatric research.*

The discussion group believed that this core competency is evaluated on MCQ examinations, such as the ABPN written certification (Part I) examination, but that it could be evaluated in a more sophisticated manner than is being done currently. Besides on cognitive examinations, this core competency could also be assessed using vignettes and under the Lifelong Learning and Self-Assessment Component of a MOC Program.

DISCUSSION OF THE EIGHTH PRACTICE-BASED LEARNING AND IMPROVEMENT CORE COMPETENCY

The eighth Practice-Based Learning and Improvement Core Competency is as follows:

8. *The physician shall demonstrate an ability to evaluate critically any relevant medical literature. This ability may include conducting and presenting reviews of current research in such formats as journal clubs, grand rounds, and/or original publications.*

This core competency was one of the few in the entire core competency outline that was thought to be at a low priority level for assessment. The discussion group clearly saw this as being evaluated under the Lifelong Learning Component of a MOC Program, perhaps through documentation of the number of reviews submitted.

DISCUSSION OF THE NINTH PRACTICE-BASED LEARNING AND IMPROVEMENT CORE COMPETENCY

The ninth Practice-Based Learning and Improvement Core Competency is as follows:

9. *The physician shall demonstrate an ability to evaluate critically any relevant medical literature. This ability may include researching and summarizing a particular problem that derives from the physician's caseload.*

This core competency was seen as being evaluated under the Lifelong Learning and Practice Assessment Components of a MOC Program. The methodology used for assessment could be the submission of case-based reports demonstrating the use of medical literature. The discussion group felt that this assessment should most probably be done by the ABPN.

DISCUSSION OF THE TENTH PRACTICE-BASED LEARNING AND IMPROVEMENT CORE COMPETENCY

The tenth Practice-Based Learning and Improvement Core Competency is as follows:

10. *The physician shall demonstrate the ability to do the following:*
    A. Review and critically assess scientific literature to determine how quality of care can be improved in relation to one's practice (e.g., reliable and valid assessment techniques, treatment approaches with established effectiveness, practice parameter adherence). Within this aim, the physician shall be able to assess the generalizability or applicability of research findings to one's patients in relation to their sociodemographic and clinical characteristics.
    B. Develop and pursue effective remediation strategies that are based on critical review of scientific literature.
    C. Learn from one's own and other specialties to improve the quality of patient care.

The discussion group saw the subpoints of this core competency as being of highest priority for assessment. They concurred that the subpoints could be assessed under the Lifelong Learning and Practice Assessment Components of a MOC Program, most likely by having diplomates present cases they had handled.

VALIDATION OF THE PRACTICE-BASED LEARNING AND IMPROVEMENT CORE COMPETENCIES

The discussion group agreed that to validate these core competencies a survey of the field would be needed with benchmarks and data outcomes, especially with functional measures for outcomes in neurology. A minor examination of the data needed would be that of how many patients a physician has cared for and how those patients have progressed to date.

SUMMARY

The full outline of the Practice-Based Learning and Improvement Core Competencies is listed below:

1. The physician shall recognize limitations in his or her own knowledge base and clinical skills, and understand and address the need for lifelong learning.
2. The physician shall demonstrate appropriate skills for obtaining up-to-date information from scientific and practice literature and other sources to assist in the quality care of patients. This shall include, but not be limited to the following:
   A. Use of medical libraries.
   B. Use of information technology, including Internet-based searches and literature databases (e.g., Medline).
   C. Use of drug information databases.
3. The physician shall demonstrate appropriate skills for obtaining up-to-date information from scientific and practice literature and other sources to assist in the quality care of patients. This shall include, but not be limited to, the active participation, as appropriate, in educational courses, conferences, and other organized educational activities both at the local and national levels.
4. The physician shall evaluate caseload and practice experience in a systematic manner. This may include case-based learning.
5. The physician shall evaluate caseload and practice experience in a systematic manner. This may include, but not be limited to, the following:
   A. Use of best practices through practice guidelines or clinical pathways.
   B. Review of patient records and outcomes.
   C. Obtaining evaluations from patients (e.g., outcomes and patient satisfaction).
6. The physician shall evaluate caseload and practice experience in a systematic manner. This may include, but not be limited to, the following:
   A. Obtaining appropriate supervision and consultation.

B. Maintaining a system for examining errors in practice and initiating improvements to eliminate or reduce errors.

7. The physician shall demonstrate an ability to evaluate critically any relevant medical literature. This ability may include using knowledge of common methodologies employed in neurological and psychiatric research.

8. The physician shall demonstrate an ability to evaluate critically any relevant medical literature. This ability may include conducting and presenting reviews of current research in such formats as journal clubs, grand rounds, and/or original publications.

9. The physician shall demonstrate an ability to evaluate critically any relevant medical literature. This ability may include researching and summarizing a particular problem that derives from the physician's caseload.

10. The physician shall demonstrate the ability to do the following:

A. Review and critically assess scientific literature to determine how quality of care can be improved in relation to one's practice (e.g., reliable and valid assessment techniques, treatment approaches with established effectiveness, practice parameter adherence). Within this aim, the physician shall be able to assess the generalizability or applicability of research findings to one's patients in relation to their sociodemographic and clinical characteristics.

B. Develop and pursue effective remediation strategies that are based on critical review of scientific literature.

C. Learn from one's own and other specialties to improve the quality of patient care.

This section of the full core competency outline was unlike the three preceding sections in that most of the core competencies herein could and should only be assessed after the physician has been in practice. The Lifelong Learning and Practice-Based Assessments of a MOC Program seemed almost to be perfectly designed for this purpose.

While most of the core competencies of this section were placed in the middle range of priority in terms of assessment, those core competencies that related to physicians understanding their own limits of knowledge and how and when to search for answers for their patients were judged of highest priority. Also in this category of highest priority for assessment was the physician's maintenance of a system for examining errors in practice and initiating improvements to eliminate or reduce those errors.

In terms of assessment methodologies for these core competencies, the discussion group decided that while some current methodologies, such as the use of cognitive examinations and vignettes might be appropriate, they stressed that such cognitive examination questions and such vignettes would have to be carefully constructed to assess what was needed here. Case-based problems might often involve the presentation of research, and there appeared to be great leeway in deciding where the responsibility for the assessments of these core competencies should rest. In some cases, specialty societies were suggested as the agents of assessment, but in other cases, the responsibility was clearly seen as that of the ABPN. In all cases, however, a critical step before any assessment could begin would be the establishment of benchmarks.

9

Professionalism Core Competencies

Alan K. Percy, M.D.

ASSUMPTIONS REGARDING THE PROFESSIONALISM CORE COMPETENCIES

The Professionalism Core Competencies, like the Interpersonal and Communications Skills Core Competencies (discussed in Chapter 7), Practice-Based Learning and Improvement Core Competencies (discussed in Chapter 8), and the Systems-Based Practice Core Competencies (discussed in Chapter 10), are regarded as core competencies which may be non-specialty specific or "generic" for most medical specialties. These "generic" core competencies stand in sharp contrast to the core competencies in the Patient Care and Medical Knowledge categories that, by their nature, must have specialty-specific components for neurology.

As discussed in Chapter 4, during the American Board of Psychiatry and Neurology (ABPN) Invitational Core Competencies Conference, six working groups were identified, and each assigned the task of discussing one of the six sections of the core competency outline. The original outline of core competencies was the result of the merging of the outlines of the six areas written by the neurology and psychiatry quadrads as convened by the American Board of Medical Specialties (ABMS) and the Accreditation Council on Graduate Medical Education (ACGME). The instructions to each working group included the recommendation to accept the basic outline unless serious changes needed to be made. Of the six working groups, only the group discussing the core competencies on professionalism found it necessary to make major changes to the outline provided. The basis for making these changes was the elimination of redundancies in the Professionalism Core Competencies.

The following summary represents the conclusions drawn regarding their amended outline. Sections deleted from the outline provided will not be discussed, as they are repetitious of the material presented here.

As the demeanor and attitudes of a physician are important in all aspects of professional life, the discussion group believed that the core competencies in the professionalism section of the outline were of highest priority for evaluation in almost all instances.

DISCUSSION OF THE FIRST PROFESSIONALISM CORE COMPETENCY

The first Professionalism Core Competency is as follows:

1. *Physicians shall demonstrate responsibility for their patients' care, including responding to communication from patients and other health professionals in a timely manner.*

The discussion group decided that this core competency could be evaluated in training and throughout practice (and especially as part of the Practice Assessment Component of the Maintenance of Certification [MOC] Program). The evaluation of this competency could be based upon an established policy for optimal physician/patient communications and on patient satisfaction surveys. Skills could be assessed before a learning intervention and then measured again afterwards.

DISCUSSION OF THE SECOND PROFESSIONALISM CORE COMPETENCY

The second Professionalism Core Competency is as follows:

2. *Physicians shall demonstrate responsibility for their patients' care, including the following:*
   A. Using medical records for appropriate documentation of the course of illness and its treatment.
   B. Providing coverage if unavailable, for example, out of town, on vacation.

The discussion group again concluded that both subpoints of this core competency could be assessed in training and throughout practice, again as part of a MOC Program. Sample medical records and peer review were suggested as methodologies of assessment. As with the previous core competency discussed above, skills could be assessed before a learning intervention and then measured again afterwards.

DISCUSSION OF THE THIRD PROFESSIONALISM CORE COMPETENCY

The third Professionalism Core Competency is as follows:

3. *Physicians shall demonstrate responsibility for their patients' care, including the following:*
   A. Coordinating care with other members of the medical and/or multidisciplinary team.
   B. Providing for continuity of care, including appropriate consultation, transfer, and termination.

While the discussion group decided that both subpoints of this core competency should be evaluated in training and throughout practice, they also thought that the first subpoint could be evaluated by oral examinations and the second subpoint both by oral and cognitive examinations.

Evaluation of how well a physician coordinates patient care with other members of the medical and/or interdisciplinary team could be handled by their peers. Data obtained from surveys or medical record review could validate this competency.

Evaluating how well a physician provides for appropriate referral or transfer when necessary could be accomplished by examining office records, medical charts, and patient satisfaction surveys. Data obtained from the above mentioned sources listed above could validate this competency.

DISCUSSION OF THE FOURTH PROFESSIONALISM CORE COMPETENCY

The fourth Professionalism Core Competency is as follows:

4. *Physicians shall demonstrate ethical behavior and personal and professional attitudes of integrity, honesty, compassion, and confidentiality in the delivery of principal or consultative patient care.*

The medical licensing bodies of each state have primary responsibility for monitoring ethical behavior in physicians. The ABPN and other ABMS member Boards rely on that measure, requiring individuals to have full, unrestricted medical licenses in order to sit for certification and recertification examinations. The discussion group also decided that ethical behavior and personal and professional attitudes of integrity, honesty, and compassion should be assessed in training and throughout practice. This assessment could be achieved through written and oral examinations such as the ABPN written certification (Part I) and oral certification (Part II) examinations and the recertification examinations, and as part of the Practice Assessment Component of the ABPN MOC Program. Patient surveys and peer reviews were suggested as methodologies of assessment. Data from such sources could also be used to validate this competency.

DISCUSSION OF THE FIFTH PROFESSIONALISM CORE COMPETENCY

The fifth Professionalism Core Competency is as follows:

5. *Physicians shall demonstrate respect for patients and colleagues as individuals, including their ages, cultures, disabilities, ethnicities, genders, socioeconomic backgrounds, religious beliefs, political leanings, and sexual orientations.*

The discussants decided that this core competency could be assessed in training and through both written and oral examinations, such as the ABPN written certification (Part I), and oral certification (Part II), and ABPN recertification examinations. For this assessment to take place as part of the current ABPN oral certification (Part II) examination, examiners would have to be trained to assure that this area would be evaluated effectively.

Again, patient surveys and peer reviews were suggested as assessment methodologies. Data from such sources could also be used to validate the competency.

DISCUSSION OF THE SIXTH PROFESSIONALISM CORE COMPETENCY

The sixth Professionalism Core Competency is as follows:

6. *Physicians shall demonstrate appreciation for end-of-life care and issues regarding provision or withholding of care.*

The discussion group thought that this core competency could be assessed using both written and oral examinations. Criteria for successful evaluation of this core competency could include examination performance, peer reviews, and assessment of how well advance directives were obtained and followed. Medical record review could aid in this assessment. Validation for this core competency could come through various outcome measures.

DISCUSSION OF THE SEVENTH, EIGHTH, AND NINTH PROFESSIONALISM CORE COMPETENCIES

The seventh, eighth, and ninth Professionalism Core Competencies, being closely related, can be discussed together. They are as follows:

7. *Physicians shall demonstrate commitment to the review and remediation of their professional conduct.*
8. *Physicians shall participate in the review of the professional conduct of their colleagues.*
9. *Physicians shall appropriately acknowledge medical errors.*

These core competencies speak to the accountability to which any professionals should hold themselves. These competencies as they relate to medical professionalism should be developed beginning in medical school, furthered in residency, and continued throughout practice life. Evaluation of these competencies can begin with faculty, program director, and peer review in medical school and residency, but their most meaningful evaluation will come as part of the Practice Assessment Component of a MOC Program.

SUMMARY

The full outline of the Professionalism Core Competencies is listed below:

1. Physicians shall demonstrate responsibility for their patients' care, including responding to communication from patients and other health professionals in a timely manner.
2. Physicians shall demonstrate responsibility for their patients' care, including the following:
   A. Using medical records for appropriate documentation of the course of illness and its treatment.
   B. Providing coverage if unavailable, e.g., out of town, on vacation.
3. Physicians shall demonstrate responsibility for their patients' care, including the following:
   A. Coordinating care with other members of the medical and/or multidisciplinary team.
   B. Providing for continuity of care, including appropriate consultation, transfer, and termination.
4. Physicians shall demonstrate ethical behavior and personal and professional attitudes of integrity, honesty, compassion, and confidentiality in the delivery of principal or consultative patient care.
5. Physicians shall demonstrate respect for patients and colleagues as individuals, including their ages, cultures, disabilities, ethnicities, genders, socioeconomic backgrounds, religious beliefs, political leanings, and sexual orientations.
6. Physicians shall demonstrate appreciation for end-of-life care and issues regarding provision or withholding of care.
7. Physicians shall demonstrate commitment to the review and remediation of their professional conduct.
8. Physicians shall participate in the review of the professional conduct of their colleagues.
9. Physicians shall appropriately acknowledge medical errors.

Discussion of the Professionalism Core Competencies at the ABPN Invitational Core Competencies Conference involved crystallizing key points of the outline and eliminating repetitious language. For all of the competencies listed above, the general consensus was that the development of professionalism is begun in medical school, continued during residency, and must be maintained throughout practice. Thus, it is important to begin instilling professional attitudes and behaviors early in medical education and to provide coaching and corrective behavior to assure that adequate standards are acquired and maintained. Initial assessment of professional behaviors and attitudes could come through specially designed cognitive questions on the written examinations, such as the ABPN certification (Part I) examination. Cognitive questions similar to those which might be used on the ABPN written certification (Part I) examination could also be included in the recertification examinations. For ongoing practice, however, the logical point of evaluation would be under the Practice-Assessment Component of the ABPN MOC Program.

As the skills that form this section of the core competency outline permeate all other sections of the outline, it would be logical that Professionalism Core Competencies be evaluated in tandem with other skills. In other words, when the Interpersonal and Communications Skills (discussed in Chapter 7) are assessed, part of that assessment could include the professionalism of the encounters. The most meaningful evaluation would emerge when the Professionalism Core Competencies are evaluated as an integral part of the other competencies.

10

Systems-Based Practice Core Competencies

H. Royden Jones, Jr., M.D. and Susan E. Adamowski, Ed.D.

DEFINING THE CATEGORY OF SYSTEMS-BASED PRACTICE CORE COMPETENCIES

The Systems-Based Practice Core Competency category is unlike any of the preceding five categories of core competencies. Physicians and laypeople alike have no trouble understanding what the terms "patient care," "medical knowledge," "practice-based learning and improvement," "interpersonal and communications skills," and "professionalism" mean. Applying these words as labels to categories of core competencies, listing the specific competencies within each category, and then deciding how and when to assess these competencies is more challenging, but generally, consensus on most points can be achieved.

The physicians who were in the Systems-Based Practice Core Competency discussion group at the Invitational Core Competencies Conference sponsored by the American Board of Psychiatry and Neurology (ABPN) in June 2001 spent a great deal of their time defining the category. Their conclusion mirrored what James E. Youker, M.D., the 28th President of the American Board of Medical Specialties (ABMS), said in his President's Column of the Summer 2001 *ABMS Record*,

> A system, as universally defined, is a set of interdependent components or elements, which interact to achieve a common purpose or goal. Physicians are familiar with the concept of scientific systems such as organ systems, but the generic meaning of the word is much broader. It encompasses the concepts of distinct entities, which function together to achieve a desired goal. Not a difficult concept, [but] why then do we find it so difficult to accept when applied to the practice of medicine as opposed to the science of medicine?

Youker explains that part of the concern may stem from the confusion between the terms "systems-based practice" and "managed care systems." He states that, "although managed care systems are inherently encompassed within the concept, the competency [category] should be envisioned in a broader context to reflect the complexities of current healthcare delivery in the United States" (Youker 2001, p. 2).

The need for serious consideration of the systems of medical practice probably stems from the 1999 Institute of Medicine report on medical errors, *To Err Is Human: Building a Safer Health System*, which lists medical mistakes as the eighth leading cause of death in the United States, ahead of deaths caused by traffic accidents, breast cancer, or AIDS. The report stresses that no one entity is to blame for the high rate of mistakes; the failure is on multiple sources. An emerging body of research exists that suggests that more often than not, "medical errors are often due to the failure of health systems rather than individual deficiencies" (Epstein and Hundert 2002, p. 226). It is primarily by improving the systems that the medical edict that promises first and foremost to "do no harm" can be actualized.

These systems of medical care are perhaps best understood as a web of interconnected services comprising physicians and other healthcare workers, hospitals and medical centers, governmental agencies, industry settings, consumers and watchdog agencies, and more. The main point to understand in regard to the Systems-Based Practice Core Competencies is that medical care is not provided in a vacuum. Most physicians do not practice alone (Randolph 1997), and even individual physicians in solo practice are enmeshed in a network of healthcare and health related agencies and entities (Frankford, Patterson, and Konrad 2000).

For example, most physicians who work with out-patients in private practice are affiliated with one or more hospitals or medical centers, and thus, they generally have an excellent working knowledge of the full realm of services available on an in-patient basis. Within the hospital network, specialists from various areas often consult with each other and function as a healthcare team. Physicians also need to be aware of the services different types of hospitals provide. Community hospitals, university-based teaching hospitals, and national centers known for specialized care have a variety of services that can be accessed, depending on patient need. To make a responsible referral, private practitioners must have a working knowledge of the hospitals or medical centers with which they are affiliated along with other related medical "systems."

The system can be broadened again when one considers that a physician in private practice must also have a full, working knowledge of community-based services for low-cost or no-cost medical care for those patients who no longer have insurance or any other means of paying for private medical care. These community-based services include far more than just medical care. These services may include housing and other social services information, addiction treatment programs like Alcoholics Anonymous or other twelve-step programs, appropriate counseling sources such as family service agencies, and the like.

To reiterate, the idea behind Systems-Based Practice Core Competencies is that physicians never practice in a vacuum. They are part of a network of programs and services available to the patient. To provide optimum healthcare, the physician must understand the full spectrum of services available. A responsible private or systems-based practitioner (e.g., a hospital-based physician) will always make available to the patient the best and most appropriate services to meet the needs of that person.

The conference group working with Systems-Based Practice Core Competencies discussed at length the longitudinal responsibility for assessing competence in this area. Competencies in this category, perhaps more than in some of the others, need to be developed incrementally over time beginning in residency and continuing throughout practice. As a corollary of their longitudinal development, longitudinal assessment is needed. The discussion group suggested that perhaps some type of mutually beneficial consortium between the residency training directors and the ABPN might be the optimum means of actualizing this for the competency assessment process.

DISCUSSION OF THE FIRST SYSTEMS-BASED PRACTICE CORE COMPETENCY

The first Systems-Based Practice Core Competency is as follows:

1. *The physician shall be able to articulate the basic concepts of systems theory and how it is used in neurology. The physician should have a working knowledge of the diverse systems involved in treating patients of all ages, and understand how to use the systems as part of a comprehensive system of care, in general, and as part of a comprehensive, individualized treatment plan.* This will include the following:
   A. Development of awareness leading to use of practice guidelines plus community, national, and allied health professional resources which may enhance the quality of life of patients with chronic neurological illnesses.
   B. Development of the ability to lead and delegate authority to healthcare teams needed to provide comprehensive care for patients with neurological diseases.
   C. Development of skills for the practice of ambulatory medicine, including time management, clinic scheduling, and efficient communication with referring physicians.
   D. Utilization of appropriate consultation and referral for the optimal clinical management of patients with complicated illnesses.
   E. Demonstration of the awareness of the importance of adequate cross-coverage.
   F. Demonstration of the awareness of the importance of accurate medical data in the communication with and effective management of patients.

The wording of the first Systems-Based Practice Core Competency is an excellent example of the comprehensiveness in wording the conference discussion group deemed necessary for each core competency in this group. The two introductory statements provide the Systems-Based Practice context for the particular core competency. The specific details of the competency are not introduced until the subpoints. This contextualization of the core competency itself into a description of what is meant by "systems" was thought to be important for the wording of these core competencies.

Point A above – the development of awareness leading to use of practice guidelines and of community, national, and allied health professional resources – is an excellent example of the longitudinal aspect of Systems-Based Practice Core Competencies. The "development of awareness" is, of necessity, a longitudinal process. This process should begin in residency (or before) and continue throughout the physician's practice life. The topics mentioned within this core competency are dynamic, not static, and it is imperative that the practicing physicians remain current with the resources available in their medical fields and systems realm.

For this reason, the discussion group suggested that assessment of this core competency begin in residency, be addressed at the time of initial certification, and be addressed again through the ABPN Maintenance of Certification (MOC) Program. Residency evaluation could be done through a variety of means depending upon the interests of and the resources available to the various residency training directors. Specific assessment methodologies during residency and practice include multiple-choice questions (MCQs), objective structured clinical examinations (OSCEs); record reviews; chart stimulated recalls; portfolio reviews; and documentation of involvement in community organizations.

Point B above – involving the leading of healthcare teams – is much less broad in scope than Point A. Point B was also judged by the discussion group to be at a lower level in terms of priority for assessment than Point A. The discussion group also saw a more narrow focus of assessment for this core competency, namely that it be assessed only through the Lifelong Learning and Practice Assessment Components of a MOC Program. Suggested evaluation methodologies included record reviews, chart stimulated recalls, portfolio, reviews, and 360-degree evaluations (evaluations done by multiple people in a person's sphere of influence, usually superiors, peers, subordinates, and patients and their families).

Like Point B, Point C – which focuses on ambulatory medicine – has a narrow focus for evaluation. The working group thought that the skills needed for the practice of ambulatory medicine, namely such skills as time management, clinic scheduling, and effective communication with referring physicians should be both taught and evaluated in residency. These same skills should then be evaluated during the Practice Assessment Component of a MOC Program.

Besides the variety of residency evaluations possible, the discussion group suggested record reviews, chart-stimulated recalls, portfolios reviews, and patient surveys as methodologies for evaluating Point C of the core competency. The group also saw this point of the core competency as being of higher priority for assessment than either of the previous points.

Similar to Point A (the development of awareness leading to the use of practice guidelines and professional resources), Point D – which discusses the role of consultation and referral – is again a broad one. The discussion group suggested wide-ranging assessment for this competency including during residency, through cognitive examinations like the ABPN written certification (Part I) and recertification examinations, through oral interviews, and through the Lifelong Learning and Practice Assessment Components of a MOC Program.

Points E and F of this core competency directly address the systems-based nature of practicing medicine. Point E, regarding cross-coverage, and Point F, regarding communication with and about patients, by their very nature, stress that the physician does not practice alone. Assessment of these competencies would need to be both wide-ranging and longitudinal.

Again, similar to what had been suggested for Point A, the discussion group suggested the following methodologies for assessment purposes of all of the other points within this competency: residency directors' attestations of competence, MCQs, oral examinations, OSCEs, record reviews, chart stimulated recalls, and portfolio reviews.

DISCUSSION OF THE SECOND SYSTEMS-BASED PRACTICE CORE COMPETENCY

The second Systems-Based Practice Core Competency is as follows:

2. *In the community system, the physician shall demonstrate the ability to recognize the limitation of healthcare resources and demonstrate the ability to act as an advocate for patients within their social and financial constraints.*

The discussion group saw the second Systems-Based Practice Core Competency as being evaluated during residency and as part of the Practice Assessment Component of a MOC Program. Suggested methodologies included residency training directors' attestations, record reviews, chart stimulated recalls, and portfolio reviews.

DISCUSSION OF THE THIRD SYSTEMS-BASED PRACTICE CORE COMPETENCY

The third Systems-Based Practice Core Competency is as follows:

3. *In the community system, the physician shall demonstrate knowledge of the resources available both publicly and privately for the treatment of neurological problems impacting a patient's ability to enjoy relationships and gain employment.*

The discussion group saw this Systems-Based Practice Core Competency as another with longitudinal parameters. Residents should begin learning about the community resources, both public and private, during their training, and then be able to transfer this ability to find and keep current with that information throughout their practice. Evaluation of this core competency for neurologists should be done during residency, during the ABPN oral certification (Part II) examination as part of initial certification, and also through the Practice Assessment Component of a MOC Program.

Suggested methodologies for this core competency included residency training directors' attestations, oral examinations, OSCEs, record reviews, chart-stimulated recalls, and portfolio reviews.

DISCUSSION OF THE FOURTH SYSTEMS-BASED PRACTICE CORE COMPETENCY

The fourth Systems-Based Practice Core Competency is as follows:

4. *In the community system, the physician shall demonstrate the ability to utilize knowledge of the legal aspects of neurological diseases as they impact patients and their families.*

Of primary importance for neurologists, this Systems-Based Practice Core Competency must be developed both longitudinally and incrementally. Residents should begin to understand the impact of the legal system on patients and their families, and upon entering practice, these physicians must keep current with both the changing laws and their changing applications and implications.

This core competency should be assessed during residency, at the time of initial certification, and through a MOC Program. Suggested methodologies include residency training directors' attestations; MCQs, such as the ABPN written certification (Part I) and recertification examinations; oral examinations, such as the ABPN oral certification (Part II) examination; OSCEs; and practice assessments.

DISCUSSION OF THE FIFTH SYSTEMS-BASED PRACTICE CORE COMPETENCY

The fifth Systems-Based Practice Core Competency is as follows:

5. *The physician shall demonstrate knowledge of and interact with managed care systems, including the following:*
   A. *Participating in utilization review communications and, when appropriate, advocating for quality patient care.*
   B. *Educating patients concerning such systems of care.*

The skills relating to this core competency should be developed in residency and assessed through the residency training directors' attestations of competency. The assessment of practicing physicians should be accomplished through the Lifelong Learning and Practice Assessment Components of a MOC Program, as appropriate to the individual specialist.

DISCUSSION OF THE SIXTH SYSTEMS-BASED PRACTICE CORE COMPETENCY

The sixth Systems-Based Practice Core Competency is as follows:

6. *The physician shall demonstrate knowledge of community systems of care and assist patients to access appropriate care and other support services. This requires knowledge of treatment settings in the community, which include ambulatory, consulting, acute care,*

partial hospital, skilled care, rehabilitation, and substance abuse facilities; halfway houses; nursing homes; and home care and hospice organizations. The physician should demonstrate knowledge of the organization of care in each relevant delivery setting and the ability to integrate the care of patients across such settings.

This Systems-Based Practice Core Competency, like some of the others discussed above, is both broad and longitudinal. The core competencies described herein can only be developed incrementally and must constantly be kept current. Training for these competencies should begin in residency and their maintenance should be continued throughout the entire practice career. Formal assessment of this core competency should come through residency training directors' attestations and OSCEs during residency; through the use of MCQs on the cognitive examinations of the ABPN written certification (Part I) and recertification examinations; through oral examinations of the ABPN oral certification (Part II) examination; and through record reviews, chart-stimulated recalls, and portfolio reviews for the Lifelong Learning and Practice Assessment Components of a MOC Program.

VALIDATION OF THE SYSTEMS-BASED PRACTICE CORE COMPETENCIES

The discussion group believed that all of the Systems-Based Practice Core Competencies could be validated by surveying the public, evaluating patient complaints, and reviewing legal records. As every core competency in this section was suggested for evaluation through the Practice Assessment Component of a MOC Program, it might become the responsibility of the ABPN to validate all of the Systems-Based Practice Core Competencies.

SUMMARY

The entire Systems-Based Practice Core Competency outline is as follows:

1. The physician shall be able to articulate the basic concepts of systems theory and how it is used in neurology. The physician should have a working knowledge of the diverse systems involved in treating patients of all ages, and understand how to use the systems as part of a comprehensive system of care, in general, and as part of a comprehensive, individualized treatment plan. This will include the following:
   A. Development of awareness leading to use of practice guidelines plus community, national, and allied health professional resources which may enhance the quality of life of patients with chronic neurological illnesses.

    B. Development of the ability to lead and delegate authority to healthcare teams needed to provide comprehensive care for patients with neurological diseases.

    C. Development of skills for the practice of ambulatory medicine, including time management, clinic scheduling, and efficient communication with referring physicians.

    D. Utilization of appropriate consultation and referral for the optimal clinical management of patients with complicated illnesses.

    E. Demonstration of the awareness of the importance of adequate cross-coverage.

    F. Demonstration of the awareness of the importance of accurate medical data in the communication with and effective management of patients.

2. In the community system, the physician shall demonstrate the ability to recognize the limitation of healthcare resources and demonstrate the ability to act as an advocate for patients within their social and financial constraints.

3. In the community system, the physician shall demonstrate knowledge of the resources available both publicly and privately for the treatment of neurological problems impacting a patient's ability to enjoy relationships and gain employment.

4. In the community system, the physician shall demonstrate the ability to utilize knowledge of the legal aspects of neurological diseases as they impact patients and their families.

5. The physician shall demonstrate knowledge of and interact with managed care systems, including the following:

    A. Participating in utilization review communications and, when appropriate, advocating for quality patient care.

    B. Educating patients concerning such systems of care.

6. The physician shall demonstrate knowledge of community systems of care and assist patients to access appropriate care and other support services. This requires knowledge of treatment settings in the community, which include ambulatory, consulting, acute care, partial hospital, skilled care, rehabilitation, and substance abuse facilities; halfway houses; nursing homes; home care; and hospice organizations. The physician should demonstrate knowledge of the organization of care in each relevant delivery setting and the ability to integrate the care of patients across such settings.

More than any of the five previous core competency sections discussed (Patient Care in Chapter 5, Medical Knowledge in Chapter 6, Interpersonal and Communications Skills in Chapter 7, Practice-Based Learning and Improvement in Chapter 8, and Professionalism in Chapter 9), this section of the core competencies outline, Systems-Based Practice, demonstrates the longitudinal character of both the development of competence and the necessity of on-going assessment.

REFERENCES

Epstein RM, Hundert EM. Defining and assessing professional competence. JAMA 2002; 287(2):226.

Frankford DM, Patterson MA, Konrad TR. Transforming practice organizations to foster lifelong learning and commitment to medical professionalism. Acad Med 2000;75:708–717.

Institute of Medicine, National Academy of Science, 1999.

Randolph L. Physician Characteristics and Distribution in the US: 1997–98 edition. Chicago, IL: Department of Data Survey and Planning. Division of Survey and Data Resources, American Medical Association, 1997.

Youker JE. The ABMS Record: What is systems-based practice? X3, p. 2, Summer 2001.

11

Cross-Competencies: What Neurologists Should Know About Psychiatry

Nicholas A. Vick, M.D., Harold P. Adams, Jr., M.D. and Thomas A. M. Kramer, M.D.

CROSS-COMPETENCY CONSIDERATIONS FOR NEUROLOGISTS

It was clear from the very beginning of the development of the American Board of Psychiatry and Neurology (ABPN) core competency outline that there would be three distinct sections for some categories of the core competencies. There would be a general section, which would discuss core competencies that both neurologists and psychiatrists would need to possess, and there would be both neurology-specific and psychiatry-specific competency sections. A basic assumption was that these specific areas would affect only the Patient Care and Medical Knowledge Core Competency Categories, and this proved true for neurology. This book focuses only on the neurological aspects of core competencies, but one area that cannot be excluded is what the Toronto discussion groups concurred that neurologists needed to know about psychiatry in terms of basic core competencies.

The reason that the ABPN came into being representing two distinct specialties is very unlike the merging of the specialties of obstetrics and gynecology to form the American Board of Obstetrics and Gynecology (ABOG) in 1930. What happened with the creation of ABOG is that what were thought to be two distinct specialties came to be seen as complementary specialties – so closely allied, in fact, that one could not practice competent obstetrics without having a complete knowledge of basic gynecology, and vice versa. Thus, it was logical that the two areas came together to form one specialty Board.

This was not the case with neurology and psychiatry. Historically, these two fields were often thought of together, especially as both were represented from the beginning in the Section on Nervous and Mental Diseases of the American Medical Association (AMA) and in some of the medical schools of the 1920s and 1930s, a single department represented both specialties. "And many clinicians, belonging to one specialty, practiced the other to a limited extent either by choice or out of economic necessity" (Hollender 1991, p. 24). Even though the specialties of neurology and psychiatry were to some extent complementary and therefore linked, the practitioners of each specialty chose to see their own specialty as separate and distinct from the other.

There were two practical reasons why the specialties of neurology and psychiatry, while electing to remain separate, still came together to form one specialty Board, the ABPN. The first was that the AMA Council on Medical Education and Hospitals and later the Advisory Board of Medical Specialties (the forerunner of the American Board of Medical Specialties) was actively working to restrict the number of specialty Boards being formed and encouraging the partnering of disciplines where possible and practical. The other reason, according to an historian of the ABPN, is that "at the time of the inception of the ABPN, there were not enough neurologists to justify the establishment of an examining board in neurology" (Forster 1960, as quoted in Hollender 1991, p. 23).

From the inception of the ABPN, examination and certification in neurology and psychiatry recognized the complementary natures of the disciplines. Initially, the same examination was given for both neurologists and psychiatrists. The examination was graded differently for the two groups of specialists, however, based on which specialty the physician had declared. Passing standards were set higher for the subject area for which one claimed professional membership than for the complementary field. Those seeking certification in both neurology and psychiatry had to meet the higher standard for both subjects on each examination.

Thus, each examination had a "major" and a "minor" section, the major section being the specialty in which certification was sought and the minor the other specialty. These "major" and "minor" sections of the certification examinations came to be known as the Part A and Part B of the ABPN Part I examination. Thus, every certified neurologist has taken and passed a "Part B" examination in psychiatry. (And the corollary is also true: every certified psychiatrist has taken and passed a "Part B" examination in neurology.)

Thus, the ABPN Core Competencies Conference held in Toronto, having representatives of both specialties present, offered a unique opportunity to document for which core competencies in psychiatry a neurologist should be held accountable (and vice versa).

Basically, the neurologists and psychiatrists attending the ABPN Invitational Core Competencies Conference agreed that psychiatrists must understand that the neurology competencies, whether they relate to anatomical pathways, neurotransmitters, medications, or basic neurophysiology, are all related to central nervous systems as opposed to peripheral nervous systems.

PSYCHIATRY-SPECIFIC PATIENT CARE CORE COMPETENCIES FOR NEUROLOGISTS

The Patient Care Core Competency discussion group felt that neurologists should be held accountable for demonstrating a comprehensive knowledge of the active and inert chemicals in drugs prescribed by psychiatrists, including their uses, side effects, and drug–drug interactions. The Patient Care Core Competency discussion group also felt that neurologists should be conversant with and have the clinical skills to elicit signs and symptoms of psychiatric origin and importance to be able to interpret their meaning and weigh them appropriately when forming differential diagnoses. Neurologists should also have the clinical skills in recognizing and managing affect, including the skills required to manage behaviorally challenging patients.

Assessment for these Patient Care Core Competencies should begin in residency training and continue throughout practice life. Depending upon when the assessment would take place, methodologies might include multiple choice questions (MCQs) on cognitive examinations, in-training evaluations, portfolios, and supervisor/peer attestations. Validation of the Patient Care Core Competencies could be made through surveys of the field.

PSYCHIATRY-SPECIFIC MEDICAL KNOWLEDGE CORE COMPETENCIES FOR NEUROLOGISTS

The Medical Knowledge Core Competency discussion group was very specific in terms of items from the psychiatry core competency outline for which neurologists should be held accountable. All of the following were listed and judged to be of the highest priority for neurologists to understand fully:

1. Human growth and development, including normal biological, cognitive, and psychosexual development.
2. Patient evaluation and treatment selection, especially the following:
   ○ Psychological testing.
   ○ Laboratory testing.
   ○ Mental status examinations.
3. Somatic treatments, including the following:
   ○ Pharmacotherapy, including the antidepressants, antipsychotics, anxiolytics, mood stabilizers, hypnotics, and stimulants, including their properties as follows:
     ▪ Pharmacological actions
     ▪ Clinical indications
     ▪ Side effects
     ▪ Drug interactions
     ▪ Toxicities
     ▪ Appropriate prescribing practices
     ▪ Cost-effectiveness
     ▪ Electroconvulsive therapy
     ▪ Light therapy
4. Emergency psychiatry, especially
   ○ Suicide prevention.
   ○ Crisis intervention.
   ○ Differential diagnoses in emergency situations.

- Treatment methods in emergency situations.
- Management of homicide, rape, and other violent behaviors.

5. Substances of abuse, including the following:
   - Pharmacological actions of substances of abuse.
   - Signs and symptoms of toxicity.
   - Signs and symptoms of withdrawal.
   - Management of toxicity and withdrawal.
   - Epidemiology, including social factors.
6. Child and adolescent psychiatry, including the following:
   - Assessment and treatment of children and adolescents.
   - Disorders usually first diagnosed in infancy, childhood, or adolescence.
   - Mental retardation and other developmental disabilities.

As with the psychiatry Patient Care Core Competencies for which neurologists should be held accountable, assessment for these Medical Knowledge Core Competencies should begin in residency training and continue throughout practice life. Depending upon when the assessment would take place, methodologies might include MCQs on cognitive examinations, in-training evaluations, portfolios, and supervisor/peer attestations. Validation of the Medical Knowledge Core Competencies could be done through surveys of the field.

It is significant to note that during the discussion, both neurologists and psychiatrists were able to agree on the neurology competencies that are necessary to the basic practice of psychiatry.

REFERENCES

Forester FM, 1960, as cited in Hollender, MH: Neurology and Psychiatry. In: The American Board of Psychiatry and Neurology: The First Fifty Years. Edited by Hollender MH. Deerfield, IL: ABPN, p. 23, 1991.

Hollender MH. Neurology and Psychiatry. In: The American Board of Psychiatry and Neurology: The First Fifty Years. Edited by Hollender MH. Deerfield, IL: ABPN, p. 24, 1991.

SECTION IV

The Impact of the Core Competencies

Section I of this book has shown how the concept of medical competence in neurology has evolved. Section II focused on two different methods of delineating core competencies: the Canadian approach of defining the roles the physician specialists play and the American approach as developed by the Accreditation Council for Graduate Medical Education and the American Board of Medical Specialties. Section III expanded upon the latter approach and discussed each of the six categories of core competencies in some detail. Section IV of this book will take the concept of core competencies from the present time into the future and attempt to predict how core competencies will affect practicing neurologists and those in training for that profession.

Chapter 12 will focus on the implications of core competencies for the purposes of initial certification through the American Board of Psychiatry and Neurology and on the evolving concept of maintenance of certification. Chapter 13 will focus on the impact that the core competencies are likely to have on the full spectrum of medical education from medical school through continuing medical education. Special emphasis will be placed on the possible role of the core competencies vis-à-vis the lifelong learning Component of the Maintenance of Certification Program. Chapter 14 will conclude this book with some educated guesses about how core competencies will affect the future practice of neurology.

Throughout this book, core competencies have been presented as fluid, living, evolving concepts, not hard and fast rules that are carved in stone. While it is likely that for residency education and certification examinations, some competencies will be made quite specific for assessment purposes, it is also likely that the methods used for assessing these core competencies will provide great latitude.

The ultimate goal of the core competencies is to provide real and realistic means for physicians to display their skills, all of which are to be used for the benefit of the patients they serve.

12

Implications of the Core Competencies on ABPN Certification and Maintenance of Certification for Neurology Practitioners

Stephen C. Scheiber, M.D. and Susan E. Adamowski, Ed.D.

ABPN CERTIFICATION AND RECERTIFICATION

From its inception, the American Board of Psychiatry and Neurology (ABPN) had as its goal the creation and administration of fair, valid, reliable certification examinations in neurology, child neurology, psychiatry, and the subspecialties. The mission of the ABPN specifies that the ultimate goal of this endeavor is to serve the public interest. The creation and administration of fair, valid, reliable examinations is an arduous process which the ABPN approaches with appropriate determination. Necessary resources of the Board have always been allocated for the accomplishment of this task.

The mission of the Board expanded with the inception of time-limited certification. The ABPN, along with its sister Boards, answered the mandate of the American Board of Medical Specialties (ABMS) by instituting certificates which expire after a given time period. Depending on the particular member Board, certificates are active for a period of six to ten years. For the ABPN, this period is ten years. As of October 1, 1994, all physicians receiving Board certification from the ABPN are issued ten-year time-limited certificates. Certificates issued in the subspecialties of addiction psychiatry, clinical neurophysiology, forensic psychiatry, geriatric psychiatry, neurodevelopmental disabilities, and pain medicine, including those issued before October 1, 1994, are also ten-year, time-limited certificates (see Note 1). What this means is that every certificate – whether for a specialty or subspecialty – that is issued by the ABPN as a time-limited certificate is active for ten years from December 31 of its year of issuance. For example, physicians who are certified in the subspecialty of addiction psychiatry on January 20, 1995, would need to recertify in addiction psychiatry before December 31, 2005 in order to have continuous certification in that subspecialty. In addition, for the physicians to be able to recertify in addiction psychiatry, their certification in general psychiatry must be current. With the exception of child and adolescent psychiatry, recertification in the relevant specialty is a prerequisite for recertification in the subspecialty.

THE CORE COMPETENCIES AND THE ABPN WRITTEN CERTIFICATION (PART I) EXAMINATION IN NEUROLOGY

The development of the written certification examination in neurology and in subspecialties begins with the examination committees writing content outlines. One major criterion for selecting committee members is their content expertise.

Content outlines are comprehensive subject area lists of topics that may be covered on the examination. The pool of examination questions covers all areas of the content outlines, but questions in all areas of the content outlines will not necessarily be on all examinations.

Of the six core competency areas (Patient Care, Medical Knowledge, Interpersonal and Communications Skills, Practice-Based Learning and Improvement, Professionalism, and Systems-Based Practice), it is proper to say that the current ABPN written certification (Part I) examination covers primarily the second competency area, Medical Knowledge and to some degree, the first competency area, Patient Care.

The physicians who attended the ABPN Invitational Core Competencies Conference in June 2001 discussed all six areas of core competencies and ascertained that while the focus of the current ABPN written certification (Part I) examination is on medical knowledge, multiple-choice questions (MCQs) *could* be written for the other core competency areas as well. It is important to note that while conference attendees stated that MCQs *could* be written for the five other core competency areas, writing valid and reliable questions in most of these subject areas could be both difficult and time-consuming. The exception here might be writing MCQs for the Systems-Based Practice Core Competency area. Even more importantly, conference attendees stressed that assessment, particularly in the four latter core competency categories, may be more effectively and efficiently accomplished using measures other than MCQs. Suggested alternative assessment measures included oral examinations, such as objective structured clinical examinations (OSCEs); portfolio review; chart-stimulated recall; peer review; and supervisor attestation.

THE CORE COMPETENCIES AND THE ABPN ORAL CERTIFICATION (PART II) EXAMINATION IN NEUROLOGY

From its inception, the ABPN realized that a written examination – no matter how comprehensive and well written – could never completely test for skills necessary for certification. To that end, an oral examination has always been required for certification in neurology. For neurology, the oral examination consists of an interview with an actual neurology patient and the interpretation of a series of neurology vignettes. The patient interview is observed by two Board-certified neurologists who are under the supervision of a senior Board-certified neurologist. The primary examiners assess the candidate's skills of interacting with the patient and then have the candidate discuss the candidate's findings including chief complaint, history of present illness and life circumstances, significant past history, review of systems, and mental status examination followed by a summary of the pertinent clinical findings. This is followed by a formulation of the case and then a differential diagnosis, a working diagnosis, prognosis, and a treatment and management plan.

The vignette component of the Part II examination is similar to the patient encounter, except that a series of short vignettes takes the place of the examination of the actual patient. Thus, obviously, the nature of the physician/patient interaction cannot be judged. Grading for the patient and the vignette portions of the Part II examination is based on the organization and presentation of data, phenomenology, diagnosis and prognosis, and etiologic, pathogenic, and therapeutic issues. The two examiners discuss their observations of each candidate and must agree on a pass or fail determination.

While the primary content emphasis of the ABPN oral certification (Part II) examination is on medical knowledge (and to a lesser extent, patient care), significant emphasis is also placed on communication skills in the patient interview and on professionalism in both the patient and vignette sections of the examination. Thus, it is accurate to say that both the core competency areas of Interpersonal and Communication Skills (discussed in Chapter 7) and Professionalism (discussed in Chapter 9) are being assessed globally with the ABPN Part II examination.

The ABPN Core Competency Committee may decide to develop and recommend to the Board a specific checklist of criteria for these two core competency areas to more evaluate formally specific competencies rather than continuing with the holistic approach.

The core competency areas of Practice-Based Learning and Improvement (discussed in Chapter 8) and Systems-Based Practice (discussed in Chapter 10) are not currently a primary focus of the ABPN oral certification (Part II) examination. It is possible that the Core Competency Committee will recommend to the Board that the Part II Examination Committee develop specific questions and/or vignettes to cover these competency areas.

It has been recognized, however, that the ABPN Part I and Part II certification examinations cannot by their very nature comprehensively evaluate all six core competency areas. One of the main conclusions of the ABPN 2001 Invitational Core Competencies Conference was that the assessment of many of the core competencies should begin early in the physician's medical education career rather than wait until the time of initial certification. This process would have many benefits. Among them may likely be the following:

- Skills, such as the manner in which a physician establishes rapport with a patient, are developed incrementally through a physician's educational and practice career. Thus, it might be appropriate to begin the assessment of such skills on an incremental basis as well. Certain levels of skills in this communications area are developed (and therefore assessable) in medical school and other levels of skills during medical residency.
- If the assessment of designated skills occurred during medical school and in residency, those not meeting criteria of success would have an excellent opportunity for remediation with the assistance of their faculty and program directors.
- Early assessment of specific competencies would allow more emphasis to be placed on the assessment of other competencies especially during the ABPN Part II certification examination. This emphasis might be placed on competencies in the Practice-Based Learning and Improvement Skills and the Systems-Based Practice Categories.

THE IMPLICATION OF CORE COMPETENCIES ON THE ABPN CERTIFICATION EXAMINATIONS

The ABPN written (Part I) and oral (Part II) certification examinations have always attempted to measure competencies necessary for successful neurology practice. The mandate of the ABMS to focus on the core competencies formalized this practice by designating six categories of competencies to be considered. The Accreditation Council for Graduate Medical Education and the ABMS facilitated the development of listing of competencies in each of the six competency areas through the work of the medical specialty quadrads (discussed in Chapter 4). The work of the ABPN Invitational Core Competencies Conference in June 2001 examined those categories especially pertinent to neurology and psychiatry, revised and added competencies as deemed necessary, and began discussion of competency assessment issues. The ABPN Core Competency Committee, appointed late in 2001, held its first meeting in January 2002.

This committee was charged with:

1. Developing an infrastructure for surveying the field, reviewing, and validating core neurology and psychiatry competencies on an on-going basis.
2. Determining which core competencies should be assessed through *traditional* ABPN certification processes and which through the ABPN Maintenance of Certification Program.

The Board will assist the committee with the integration of the core competencies into the field by having discussions with appropriate institutions and organizations.

Thus, it is both correct and appropriate to say that the introduction of core competencies into the certification work of the ABPN has not substantially changed the vision of the Board, but instead the core competencies have provided a structured format for achieving the mission of the Board. The ultimate goal, serving the American public by providing the means of certifying neurologists, has become more structured and more formalized.

The core competencies, when fully integrated into the course of medical education and residency and when correlated with the ABPN written and oral certification examinations, should provide a comprehensive structure for the initial assessments of physician competencies.

The core competencies structure, especially by delineating competencies in the area of Practice-Based Learning and Improvement and in the area of Systems-Based Practice, points out the necessity for more than initial certification.

RECERTIFICATION'S EVOLUTION INTO A MAINTENANCE OF CERTIFICATION PROGRAM

Chronologically parallel with the development of the core competencies structure came the realization on the part of the ABMS that even the recertification of physicians on a periodic basis was not sufficient to maintain the public trust. The public both demanded and deserved to know that their physicians maintained a level of competence that was more than what could be shown by the successful completion of a day-long written examination in neurology every ten years.

To this end, the ABMS developed its four-part Maintenance of Certification (MOC) Program©, into which the written recertification examination has since been subsumed. The four parts of the MOC Program© include the following:

1. Evidence of Professional Standing.
2. Evidence of Lifelong Learning and Periodic Self-Assessment.
3. Evidence of Cognitive Expertise.
4. Evidence of Evaluation of Practice Performance.

All twenty-four member Boards of the ABMS were directed to implement a Maintenance of Certification Program suitable for their diplomates.

THE CORE COMPETENCIES AND THE ABPN MOC PROGRAM

Core competencies clearly relate to all four elements of the ABPN MOC Program. In some cases, one category of core competencies clearly and/or primarily relates to one of the elements of the ABPN MOC Program. For example, the requirement for licensure, handled by state licensing bodies and not the ABPN, clearly relates to the category of Professionalism Core Competencies. While it would *not* be correct to say that every licensed physician has met all of the competencies within the Professionalism Category, it would be correct to assume that unlicensed physicians are seriously deficient enough in the area of Professionalism that they do not merit continued certification.

The second element of the ABPN MOC Program – evidence of periodic self-assessment and documentation of lifelong learning – relates most directly to the Practice-Based Learning and Improvement Core Competency area. The relationship between this element of the ABPN MOC Program and the above-named core competency category will be developed from recommendations the ABPN MOC Committee makes to the full ABPN Board. The ABMS has directed its member Boards that this component of each Board's Maintenance of Certification Program must be satisfied according to the dictates of the individual member Boards before physicians can be admitted to sit for the recertification examination.

Various ABMS member Boards have begun delineating requirements to document lifelong learning. Physician learning after residency has traditionally been measured in units of continuing medical education (CME) credits. While some ABMS member Boards will continue to use CME credits as a measure of lifelong learning, it is anticipated that a better system, which reflects educational efforts that will improve practice will be developed for those wishing to recertify through the ABPN. As this process is developed and formalized, it will be communicated by traditional methods, such as the ABPN *Annual Report* published in the *American Journal of Psychiatry*, as well as newer means, such as the ABPN *Diplomate* newsletter and on the ABPN website (www.abpn.com).

The third element of the ABPN MOC Program – evidence of cognitive expertise – will be handled for neurologists through the ABPN recertification examinations. The ABMS mandates that these be secure, proctored examinations, and, as stated earlier, evidence of self-assessment and lifelong learning must be documented prior to the administration of such examinations. It is anticipated that recertification examinations will be closely modeled on the ABPN written certification (Part I) examinations, but with primary focus on applications to practice rather than on basic sciences.

The ABPN Board of Directors has instructed the ABPN MOC Committee to focus their initial efforts on the first three elements of the MOC Program as discussed above. The fourth element of the ABPN MOC Program – the assessment of practice performance – will be implemented last. As this entire assessment becomes formalized, details will be communicated through the various media described above.

THE IMPLICATIONS OF CORE COMPETENCIES ON THE ABPN MAINTENANCE OF CERTIFICATION PROGRAM

The ABPN supports the mandate of the ABMS to evolve the recertification examination into a MOC Program©. Regarding the ABPN's progress toward implementing the four elements of the MOC Program, the following can be said:

1. Regarding evidence of professional standing, the ABPN foresees no major change in its current procedure of requiring a full, unrestricted medical license at the time of registration for the administration of the recertification examination.
2. The ABPN Maintenance of Certification Committee will establish acceptable procedures for the documentation of self-assessment and lifelong learning on the part of individual physicians prior to their registration for the recertification examination. It is likely that this effort will be carried out in cooperation with relevant professional specialty societies.
3. The ABPN will model its recertification examinations on the MCQ format of the ABPN written certification (Part I) examination. The recertification examination will focus on the core competencies as they apply to physicians in practice. Only physicians who have met the two criteria listed above will be able to register for the recertification examination. All recertification examinations will be given on computer.
4. The last part of the ABPN MOC Program to be implemented will be the assessment of performance in practice. The MOC Committee will be responsible for this procedure and making recommendations to the Board.

All aspects of the ABPN MOC Program will be discussed in the ABPN *Diplomate* newsletter and on the ABPN website (www.abpn.com).

NOTES

1. Ten-year time-limited certification for child and adolescent psychiatry began in 1995.

13

Implications of the Core Competencies on the Full Spectrum of Medical Education for Clinical Neurology Practice: From Medical School Through Continuing Medical Education

Thomas A. M. Kramer, M.D.

FROM TIME-BASED TO COMPETENCY-BASED MEDICAL EDUCATION

It would be difficult to overstate the potential impact on medical education in general – and on neurology education in particular – of the core competency movement. The shift toward basing education on the acquisition of specific competencies as opposed to time-limited rotations represents a sea change, the likes of which probably have not been seen since the institution of the Flexner Report, which precipitated the transition from apprentice-based medical training to curriculum-based medical training.

Medical education as a whole remains a time-driven enterprise. It takes four full-time years to graduate from an American medical school. Graduate medical education has specific lengths of residency training ranging from three to seven years depending on the specialty selected. Continuing medical education is measured in hours. Even the most intriguing educational experiment in medicine is done by altering the sequence of events still within prescribed time frames or, at most, combining and condensing time frames while providing the opportunity for continuity experiences in the case of combined training programs. It is only with the core competency movement that the possibility exists that endurance for a specific period of time will not be the primary criterion for the completion of medical training.

This is not to say that there are not already some competency measures in place within the medical education system as it currently exists. Medical students are graded with at least pass/fail grades – if not letter grades – in their preclinical courses and their clinical rotations. They must pass these if they are to proceed. They also have exams, such as the United States Medical Licensing Examination Steps, that most schools require for promotion and graduation. Graduate medical education has fewer competency-based assessments required for its completion, and these vary from specialty to specialty and from program to program. More than medical school, these assessments remain driven primarily by spending the requisite number of months and years doing required rotations. Continuing medical education in its current form is driven almost exclusively by time. Although much continuing medical education has pre- and post-assessments of the material presented, these assessments usually have little to do with the granting of credit. If physicians sit through the program, they earn the continuing medical education credit. Thus, there is a spectrum in which competency is assessed somewhat in medical school, less so in graduate medical education, and even less so in continuing medical education.

IMPLICATIONS OF THE CORE COMPETENCIES FOR MEDICAL SCHOOLS

In medical schools, the impact of core competencies has already begun to be felt to a certain extent. Since many schools have comprehensive exams – particularly between preclinical and post-clinical training – and students cannot proceed to the next phase unless they pass the exam, there is already some sense that at least this part of medical education requires some documentation of competency. Still, most clinical rotations are time-driven, and successful completion of training is not competency-based in most institutions. Medical school, however, remains the only institution within the sequence of medical education that seems to, at the present time, routinely require the demonstration of competency for promotion. It is also the institution that, in a functional sense, is most likely to adapt smoothly to the competency paradigm. With the diminution – if not the elimination – of time as the important criterion for medical education, the question is then begged whether different students can proceed through training at different rates of speed, thus making the length of medical school variable. If a medical student achieves competency in all the things necessary to complete a program sooner rather than later, could that student graduate sooner rather than later? Since medical students pay tuition to attend school, it is perhaps possible that someone who attains all the core competencies early could graduate early and thus save some tuition fees. Conversely then, it would also be possible that those students who are unable to attain all competencies within the prescribed time could attend school longer, continuing to pay tuition for the privilege, until they have achieved competence in all competencies necessary for graduation. Medical students offset their cost to the institution at least to a certain extent, and, for the most part, are not required members of the healthcare team. For all these reasons, shorter or longer courses of training are easier for a medical school to adapt to, and, as such, medical student education may be the most flexible of the different medical education institutions in the transition to a core competencies model.

IMPLICATIONS OF THE CORE COMPETENCIES FOR RESIDENCY PROGRAMS

The application of core competencies to the graduate medical education system, however, initially appears to be considerably more problematic. While one can make the argument that the acquisition of competencies is even more crucial for a resident in specialty training, residents under the current system are funded for a specific number of years and are needed by many of the hospitals that employ them to do specific tasks for given periods of time. Rotations within a residency-training program are similar to a musical chairs game with the same number of chairs at all times. When someone moves from one chair to another, there must be someone to fill the vacant chair and someone must give up a chair for the first person to sit in. If residents take longer or shorter periods of time to finish their training, funding formulas and clinical coverage at the training institution will be affected. For those residents who require longer to attain the core competencies, there may not be funding, as least under the current system, for them to train for a longer period of time. Similarly, if residents are able to attain the required competencies in a shorter period of time, the program may still need them present for the originally agreed upon duration to be able to cover clinical service with the requisite number of physicians.

IMPLICATIONS OF THE CORE COMPETENCIES FOR CONTINUING MEDICAL EDUCATION

Continuing medical education will also be changed dramatically by core competencies. There has been a great deal of criticism of the current continuing medical education system, in terms of conflicts of interest by providers funded by pharmaceutical companies, the lack of meaningful assessment of the programs and the physicians participating in them, and the relevance to practice of program content. Since all members of the American Board of Medical Specialties (ABMS) are moving to time-limited certificates, physicians will be required in some way to demonstrate competency at least sporadically. The institution of a Maintenance of Certification (MOC) Program by the ABPN dovetails well with the core competency movement in that it will require physicians on an ongoing basis to educate themselves, document the efficacy of that education, and demonstrate in some way that they are applying that education in the form of competent practice. There is very little controversy that physicians need ongoing education in order to maintain and increase their knowledge and skills. Core competencies, when promulgated and assessed, will hopefully make this process more structured and more meaningful.

ADDITIONAL ISSUES; POSSIBLE SOLUTIONS

The general issue of time versus competency in the completion of any medical training program remains to be resolved. It is probably true that it will be necessary for training programs to have a combination of competency assessment and prescribed lengths of time at least within guidelines. This may be necessary not just for smooth functioning of the training programs, but also for the utility of requiring at least a minimum of time in training services to get a sense of the culture of those services beyond the acquisition of core competencies.

Most of the current discussion concerning the transition to a core competency-driven educational system has centered on what the core competencies will be, who will write them, and what kind of latitude the various training programs will have with them. These concerns may be, to a certain extent, missing the point. Change is fundamental to the practice of quality medicine. Treatments are continuously improving. The understanding of health and disease issues continues to expand. Any kind of rigidity in the determination of what core competencies are threatens to be a regressive force that will lead to progressively obsolete competencies. Infrastructures need to be developed under which core competencies can be continually modified to stay current with the field. These changes need to occur throughout the entire spectrum of medical education, as medical students need to be given the most current information and skills, residents need to be taught to practice using the most recently developed treatments, and practicing physicians need to be kept up to date with the constant changes. The challenge will be for the accrediting bodies to develop a mechanism to revise the required competencies in some ongoing fashion, perhaps in ways similar to the manner in which certification Boards continually update their exams.

Far and away the most difficult challenge of the institution of core competencies to the medical education infrastructure is the development of appropriate assessment methodologies for all the competencies. Medical education has been traditionally dependent on multiple-choice question (MCQ) exams. While these examinations are enormously effective in assessing medical knowledge and somewhat effective in determining abilities in patient care, there are many parts of the six general categories of core competencies that cannot be assessed with such examinations. For example, the efficacy of communication, the establishment of rapport with a patient, and issues of professionalism do not lend themselves easily to assessment through MCQs.

Many certification Boards give oral examinations to increase their assessment abilities, and medical schools are moving toward both actual patient examinations and oral examinations as a way to assess their students. Other evaluation methodologies, such as computer based testing with vignettes and MCQs, portfolio assessments, and other standardized clinical scenarios are in various phases of development. It is relatively easy to develop a list of competencies that one would want a particular physician to have. It is considerably more difficult to find reliable and valid methods to assess whether that physician is indeed competent in those areas. The extent to which the medical education establishment rises to this particular challenge will for the most part determine the success or failure of core competencies in medical education.

14

A Forward View: Core Competencies in Future Neurology Practice

Stephen C. Scheiber, M.D., Thomas A. M. Kramer, M.D., and Susan Adamowski, Ed.D.

Predicting the future is always an impossible task. Any discussion of the future impact of core competencies on clinical practice in neurology should only be intended to provoke discussion, thought, and flexibility. Very few authors – if any – have had any success in predicting the direction in which healthcare in general will go. The many variables involved and the many unforeseen influences that have had a profound impact on the provision of healthcare create overwhelming odds that any predictions made in this chapter will probably seem short-sighted in the years to come.

There are, however, some current general trends in healthcare. The future of these trends will probably be the primary determinants of the impact of core competencies on clinical practice. One current trend is a move toward more competition among healthcare providers, probably on the institutional level and perhaps even on the individual practitioner level. This appears to be where the managed care revolution is leading. If healthcare decision-making is going to be increasingly driven by marketing issues, then there will be a push toward concrete aspects that can be advertised as positive aspects of care. One can, for instance, easily note the increased number of commercials on television and in print describing hospital systems or healthcare organizations as places where consumers would receive optimum care.

As a result of this marketing, Board certification of the physicians within given systems may become increasingly common. As a corollary to hospitals advertising their Board-certified neurologists, neurologists in private practice might market themselves as being Board-certified. One possible outcome of this trend is that there will be increased public awareness of the meaning of Board certification. In 1999, the American Board of Psychiatry and Neurology did a series of focus groups with consumers of neurology and psychiatry care. Focus group participants had virtually no knowledge of the meaning of the term "Board certification."

One might anticipate the meaning and the importance of Board certification increasing through marketing enterprises already under way.

If public awareness of Board certification increases and Board certification becomes associated with the satisfactory demonstration of core competencies as described earlier in this book, then core competencies as defined and assessed have at least the potential to become *the* central issue in healthcare. Practitioners will need to be able to demonstrate competency in order to attract and retain patients. Competition among providers will create marketing that will educate consumers so that they will demand proficiency in core competencies in the physicians that they consult for healthcare.

Core competencies, as they are integrated into graduate medical education, have been described as hurdles for the physician in training to get past. The transition, as described previously, between spending a certain amount of time in training as the primary determinant of competency versus actually demonstrating identified competencies should more appropriately be described as a series of "checkpoints" in training. Some physicians in training will proceed easily through these training checkpoints, and others will be held back until they obtain the specified competency. This process may initially reduce the flow of physicians in training from becoming full practitioners.

One example of this phenomenon is occurring now with the Educational Commission for Foreign Medical Graduates (ECFMG) clinical skills assessment examination. International medical graduates (IMGs) constitute a large group of physicians practicing in this country. In particular, they constitute a large group of the graduate medical education population. The ECFMG is now requiring that IMGs pass a clinical skills assessment examination (CSA) using standardized patients before they can enter approved residency training programs in this country. The CSA provides IMGs with the opportunity to demonstrate their ability to interact with patients and make basic clinical decisions. Preliminary data from the ECFMG indicates that the CSA examination serves as an excellent means of assuring the IMGs have skill levels that will allow them to compete in the American residency program. The CSA examination effectively creates a set of core competencies for IMGs. Those who do not demonstrate that they have achieved the necessary competencies are unable to enter into the US medical education system. As more core competencies are integrated into medical education and assessments are developed for them, it is likely that this trend will continue.

The major impact of core competencies on clinical practice for the future is likely to be enormously positive. The reason for this is that core competencies can provide the healthcare system with a level of quality control it has never had – at least as far as physician competence is concerned. Currently, most people locate doctors by consulting lists in health insurance books or by having doctors recommended to them by a friend or another physician. There is currently no objective way to ascertain if a physician is professionally competent. The core competency system has the potential to allow patients to approach the healthcare system with a great deal more confidence that their doctors are competent and able to perform their duties. The trend towards demedicalizing a great deal of healthcare may also reverse itself as physician's assistants, nurse practitioners, and neurologists are unable to demonstrate the delineated physician core competencies. Core competencies, as defined, would make it very clear exactly what physicians are trained to do and which tasks are inappropriate for non-physicians.

One major problem in current healthcare is the limited extent to which practicing physicians are monitored. With core competencies integrated into Maintenance of Certification Programs©, physicians who are unable or unwilling to keep up with their fields will not be able to demonstrate on-going competency and will be eliminated from practice. In medicine, the wisdom of age is often counterbalanced by the lack of new knowledge. Core competencies would reassure patients that their senior physicians are keeping up to date and also counteract the trend that younger doctors tend to be more current than older ones. It is easy to say that all doctors should keep up with their field. Core competencies provide a system, an infrastructure, to ensure that.

To reiterate, it is very difficult to predict the future. The impact of core competencies on clinical practice very much remains to be seen. It is safe to predict, however, that the effect of core competencies on future practice will be both profound and positive. Implementation of core competencies into physician training and into Maintenance of Certification Programs© should lead to the overall improvement of healthcare.

Neurology Quadrad Outline of Core Competencies

PATIENT CARE

1. Neurology residents must be able to provide scientifically based, comprehensive and effective diagnosis and management for patients with neurologic disease. Residents are expected to master the following skills and abilities by completion of training:

Clinical Skills

- Elicit a complete neurologic history from adults and children using collateral history if necessary
- Perform an appropriate general and neurologic examination
- Determine whether a patient's symptoms and signs are the result of organic or psychologic disease and provide localization of possible organic pathologies
- Generate a rational formulation, differential diagnosis, laboratory investigation and management plan

Technical Skills

- Lumbar puncture, tensilon and caloric testing
- Identify plain films, myelography, angiography, CT, isotope, MRI and PET/SPECT imaging of the neuroaxis
- Evaluate the application and relevance of investigative procedures and their interpretation in the diagnosis of neurologic disease including electroencephalogram, motor and sensory nerve conduction studies, electromyography, evoked potentials, polysomnography, electronystagmogram, audiometry, perimetry, psychometry, CSF analysis, and radiographic studies as outlined above
- Identify and describe gross and microscopic specimens taken from the normal nervous system and from patients with major neurologic disorders.

2. Recognize and treat potentially life-threatening neurologic disorders.
3. Evaluate, assess and recommend cost-effective management of patients with neurologic symptoms and disease.

Medical Knowledge

1. Neurology residents must be able to demonstrate knowledge and understanding of the pathophysiology of major neurologic and psychiatric disorders and be familiar with the specific basis of neurologic disease as outlined and regularly updated by the American Board of Psychiatry and Neurology including:
   A. neuroanatomy
      1. cerebral cortex
      2. connecting systems
      3. basal ganglia/thalamus
      4. brainstem
      5. cerebellum
      6. cranial nerves
      7. spinal cord
      8. spinal roots/peripheral nerves
      9. ventricular system/CSF pathways
      10. vascular
      11. neuromuscular junction/muscles
      12. autonomic nervous system
      13. embryology
      14. pain pathways
      15. radiologic anatomy/cerebral blood vessels (angio or MRA)
   B. neuropathology
      1. basic patterns of reaction
      2. cerebrovascular disease
      3. trauma (cranial and spinal)
      4. metabolic/toxic/nutritional diseases
      5. infections
      6. demyelinating diseases/leukodystrophies
      7. neoplasms
      8. congenital/developmental disorders
      9. degenerative/heterodegenerative disorders
      10. myopathies
      11. peripheral nerve disorders
      12. radiologic pathology pertinent to assigned pathology sections
   C. neurochemistry
      1. carbohydrate metabolism
      2. lipid metabolism
      3. protein metabolism
      4. neurotransmitters

     5. axonal transport
     6. energy metabolism
     7. blood–brain barrier
     8. biochemistry of membranes/receptors/ion channels
     9. neuronal excitation
    10. vitamins (general aspects)
    11. inborn errors of metabolism
    12. electrolytes and minerals
    13. neurotoxins
    14. free radical scavengers
    15. excitotoxicity
D. neurophysiology
     1. basic
       a. membrane physiology
       b. synaptic transmission
       c. sensory receptors and perception
       d. special senses
       e. reflexes
       f. segmental and suprasegmental control of movement
       g. cerebellar function
       h. reticular system/mechanisms of sleep and arousal/consciousness/circadian rhythms
       i. rhinencephalon/limbic system/the visceral brain
       j. learning and memory
       k. cortical organizations and function
       l. pathophysiology of epilepsy
      m. cerebral blood flow
      n. autonomic function
      o. blood–brain barrier
     2. clinical
       a. EEG
       b. evoked responses
       c. EMG/nerve conduction studies
       d. sleep studies
E. neuropharmacology
     1. anticonvulsants
     2. antibiotics/antimicrobials/vaccines
     3. antioxidants
     4. neuromuscular agents
     5. antidyskinesia drugs (including antiparkinsonians)
     6. vitamins (clinical aspects)
     7. analgesics (non-narcotics, narcotics, and other centrally active agents)
     8. anticoagulants/antiplatelets/thrombolytic agents
     9. hormones

10. autonomic agents
11. anticholinesterase drugs
12. neurologic side effects of systemic drugs
13. miscellaneous drugs
F. neuroimmunology/neurovirology
    1. molecular pathogenesis of multiple sclerosis
    2. molecular neurology of prion diseases and slow viruses
    3. immunology in MS/MG/other neurologic disorders
G. neurogenetics/molecular neurology and neuroepidemiology
    1. Mendelian-inherited diseases
    2. mitochondrial disorders
    3. trinucleotide repeat disorders
    4. channelopathies
    5. genetics of epilepsy
    6. molecular genetics of brain tumors
    7. other genetic disorders/mechanisms
    8. ischemic penumbra
    9. molecular approaches to stroke therapy
    10. polymerase chain reaction
    11. risk factors in neurologic disease
    12. demographics of neurologic disease
H. neuroendocrinology
I. neuroimaging
    1. plain skull/spine radiology
    2. MRI/MRV/MRA
    3. CT scan
    4. CT myelography
    5. Angiography
    6. SPECT/PET
J. neuro-ophthalmology
    1. vision and visual pathways
    2. visual fields
    3. pupils
    4. ocular motility
    5. fundi/retina/optic nerve
K. neuro-otology
    1. hearing/auditory function and testing
    2. vertigo/vestibular function and testing
L. cerebrospinal fluid
    1. normal CSF constituents and volume
    2. pathologic CSF patterns
        a. cellular
        b. chemical
        c. enzymatic
        d. serologic
M. critical care and emergency neurology

    N. geriatric neurology

    O. headache and facial pain

    P. interventional neurology

    Q. movement disorders

    R. neurological rehabilitation

2. Demonstrate the ability to reference and utilize electronic information systems to access medical, scientific and patient information.

INTERPERSONAL AND COMMUNICATION SKILLS

1. Neurology residents must be able to counsel fellow physicians, patients and families regarding diagnostic and therapeutic options for the effective management of neurologic symptoms and disorders with specific regard to:
   * Interdisciplinary care and involvement of allied health professionals
   * Genetic counseling and palliative care when appropriate
   * Consideration and compassion for the patient in providing accurate medical information and prognosis.
2. Neurology residents must demonstrate interpersonal skills and documentation habits needed for effective communication with fellow physicians, patients, families and allied health professionals including:
   * Effective listening
   * Use of informed consent when ordering investigative procedures
   * Maintenance of accurate, timely and legible medical records.
3. Neurology residents must be able to counsel patients and others about the prevention of neurologic disorders, including risk factors, genetic and environmental concerns.

PRACTICE-BASED LEARNING AND IMPROVEMENT

Neurology residents must be able to investigate and evaluate their patient care practices, appraise and assimilate scientific evidence and improve their patient care practices. Residents are expected to demonstrate skill in the following areas:

* Case-based learning
* Use of best practices through practice guidelines or clinical pathways
* Participation in quality assurance and improvement
* Collection and analysis of patient data

PROFESSIONALISM

Neurology residents must demonstrate a commitment to carrying out professional responsibilities, adherence to ethical principals, and sensitivity to a diverse patient population. Residents are expected to:

* Demonstrate personal and professional attitudes of integrity, honesty and compassion in the delivery of principal or consultative patient care

- Regularly review one's own skills and knowledge, realize limitations and respond to others' evaluation of one's own professional performance
- Demonstrate a commitment to excellence in clinical practice through the establishment of lifelong learning habits and continuing medical education
- Demonstrate respect for patient's cultural, ethnic, religious and socioeconomic background in providing patient care
- Demonstrate appreciation of end-of-life care and issues regarding provision or withholding of care

SYSTEMS-BASED PRACTICE

Neurology residents must be trained to recognize they are part of a large and intricate health system that has many implications for their ability to care for patients and, more importantly, impact upon their patient's human needs and financial resources. This broad awareness of the context in which neurologists practice, beyond diagnosis and treatment planning, requires competence in seven areas:

- Recognize the limitation of resources for healthcare and demonstrate the ability to act as an advocate for patients within their social and financial constraints
- Willingness to participate in utilization review and comply with documentation requirements in medical records
- Develop awareness of practice guidelines, community, national and allied health professional resources which may enhance the quality of life of patients with chronic neurological illness
- Develop the ability to lead and delegate authority to healthcare teams needed to provide comprehensive care for patients with neurologic disease
- Develop skills for the practice of ambulatory medicine including time management, clinic scheduling and efficient communication with referring physicians
- Utilize appropriate consultation and referral for the optimal clinical management of patients with complicated medical illness
- Demonstrate awareness of the importance of adequate cross-coverage and availability of accurate medical data in the communication with and efficient management of patients under their care.

Index